Kim Embrey
Coca and the Victorians

Histoire | 244

Kim Embrey, born in 1991, is a secondary school teacher of English, bilingual geography, and ethics in southern Germany. As a historian, she did her doctorate at Goethe-Universität Frankfurt am Main and is the secretary of the German Association for British Studies. She is an active member of several international academic societies, including the Royal Historical Society, the Britain and the World Society, and the Alcohol and Drugs History Society. Her research interests lie at the intersection of British sociocultural, scientific, and medical history.

Kim Embrey

Coca and the Victorians

From Botanical Curiosity to Regulated Drug, 1835-1912

[transcript]

D.30

Bibliographic information published by the Deutsche Nationalbibliothek
The Deutsche Nationalbibliothek lists this publication in the Deutsche Nationalbibliografie; detailed bibliographic data are available in the Internet at https://dnb.dnb.de

Hermannstraße 26 | D-33602 Bielefeld | live@transcript-verlag.de

Cover design: Lena Schäfferling based on a design by Kim Embrey
Cover illustration: Photo by Laszlo Mates at istockphoto.com (1031592512), modified
Printing: Elanders Waiblingen GmbH, Waiblingen
Print-ISBN: 978-3-8376-7977-9 | PDF-ISBN: 978-3-8394-4419-1
ISSN of series: 2702-9409 | eISSN of series: 2702-9417

Printed on permanent acid-free text paper.

For R

–

May love and the pursuit of wisdom accompany you
from the moment you open your eyes for the first time until you take your last breath.

Contents

Acknowledgements

I would like to express my deepest gratitude to my supervisor and mentor Prof Dr Torsten Riotte who trusted in my abilities from the very beginning and who provided valuable feedback over the last two-and-a-half years, no matter where I was in the world. Your continuous support was not self-evident, and I appreciated any comment or criticism that contributed to me reaching my goal – even if that meant removing 40 pages. Our scholarly exchange has greatly fostered my critical thinking and helped me to think outside the box. Thank you from the bottom of my heart.

This endeavour would also not have been possible without the generous support from the German Historical Institute London that awarded me with a scholarship which enabled me to conduct research in British archives and libraries, and which also facilitated the expansion of my academic network.

I also want to thank my favourite teacher colleagues, who probably thought I was insane to add more workload to my full-time job as a teacher, but who provided important moral support.

Many thanks should also go to my parents who believed in me ever since I was little and who supported me in chasing my dreams. It was not always easy, but it was definitely worth it. Special thanks go to my sister Nina whose creativity and artistic talent never seize to amaze me.

Last but not least, I am beyond thankful for my husband, Michael, who eventually tipped the scale for me to pursue my PhD and transferred me his scholarship to expand my historical knowledge. His support, encouragement, and belief in me throughout this journey has been a constant source of strength. I feel blessed that our genuine interest in history is mutual and I am lucky to share this life with you.

Introduction

> The history of coca is that of many other drugs -- known at first to few, and confined to limited areas, then described more or less intelligently by some learned inquirer, and after a time introduced into all parts of the world, and finally, when applied to legitimate uses, adding to the conveniences and pleasures of life, and becoming instead of a curiosity the prized possession of millions.[1]

How Alfred J H Crespi, a member of the Royal College of Physicians, summarized the history of coca in just one sentence in 1889 might at first glance make sense to readers unacquainted with the history of narcotics in the nineteenth century but there is much more to the (hi)story that he could not yet have anticipated. Take, for example, the negative consequences for public health, the spread of its illegitimate use and the evolving problem with addiction, and the political restrictions that eventually involved several nations across the globe. The history of coca encompassed many more aspects that made it an exceptional narcotic in the long nineteenth century rather than a tag-along of the ever-present opium, and today it has just sparked renewed interest of politicians and researchers alike.

During the recent 68th session of the Commission on Narcotic Drugs at the United Nations Conference in Vienna in spring 2025, Columbia and Bolivia jointly requested coca to be removed from the list of narcotics after more than 113 years. This raises questions as to why coca was restricted in the 1912 International Opium Conference in The Hague in the first place. Back then, the plant gained notoriety for being the raw material for the manufacturing of cocaine although it had been used by the native populations of South America for millennia without the devastating effects of the purified product known today.

1 Alfred J H Crespi, "Some recent scientific Advances," *The Gentleman's Magazine* (October 1889), 399.

This circumstance requires a revisiting and renegotiating of coca in Victorian Britain before it became an illegal and internationally restricted narcotic.

When it arrived in Britain in the mid-nineteenth century, coca was an exotic novelty, though not the first narcotic that enjoyed widespread popularity among Victorians. For decades, Britain had already held the monopoly over the opium trade in Asia and ensured its continuance through two Opium Wars between 1839 and 1860. Today, opium is one of the most well-researched commodities in British history, particularly as a colonial product, and thus has been the preeminent narcotic in the nineteenth century history of narcotics.[2] This bias has existed for quite some time but neglected other narcotics, such as coca, whose introduction into the British and the European market in general laid the foundation for their global careers in the twentieth century. Therefore, it makes for an interesting investigation whether coca also became a colonial product for Britain and how its career differed to or resembled that of opium.

This book examines how the Victorians reacted to coca as a novelty in the medicinal scene, as it was considered a breakthrough in Central Europe, and under which circumstances the British tried to make it a colonial commodity of their own in the nineteenth century. It is embedded in a nexus of cultural, economic, political, and medicinal aspects that contribute to its exceptional role in the history of drugs in Britain. This approach allows for making interdependencies more visible since it is impossible to examine narcotics consumption without their mode of cultivation, the trade that provides them, the political decision-making that accompanies it, and the people at the end of the chain who have their own reasons to indulge in the habit. Looking at those circumstances is important as drug consumption today is still stigmatised regardless of historical circumstances.[3] Coca, although not the most popular narcotic in nineteenth-century Britain, experienced a short-lived career cycle that evolved from the fascination accompanying its introduction to its global prohibition for other than medicinal purposes within just fifty years. As South American

2 A noted work here is certainly Virginia Berridge and Griffith Edwards, *Opium and the People* (London, New York: St. Martin's Press, 1987) but more recent works include Martin Booth, *Opium: A History* (London: Simon & Schuster Ltd., 1996), Thomas Dormandy, *Opium – Reality's Dark Dream* (New Haven: Yale University Press, 2012), and Amitav Ghosh, *Smoke and Ashes* (London: John Murray, 2024).

3 Compare, for example, David T Courtwright, *Forces of Habit* (Cambridge: Harvard University Press, 2001) and minutes of the Commission on Narcotic Drugs at the United Nations Conference in Vienna 2023.

countries had already argued at the United Nations Drug Conference in Vienna in March 2023, it is time to revisit and renegotiate the history of coca to make a distinction between the Incan leaf and the narcotic that has immensely contributed to the illegal drug trade in the twentieth and twenty-first century.[4]

In this book, I focus on the history of coca between 1835 when coca was first mentioned in a British publication called *Hooker's Botanical Companion*, and 1912 when the International Opium Convention in The Hague made coca a globally restricted narcotic which could only be used for medicinal purposes. This time frame is significant for the history of coca since it traces its status and history before the drug's introduction into the British market, as well as the circumstances of it becoming a popular and eventually, restricted narcotic. It also helps to compare coca's career to that of opium which experienced its heyday during the Victorian Era and allows for a comparison with the reaction to coca in other European countries. After all, this temporal limitation enables a richer understanding of the history of coca in Britain. Due to spatial limitations, I do not discuss the career of cocaine in the twentieth and twenty-first century here. Similarly, the history of coca in South American countries at the same time are neglected although occasional references to the treatment of coca there during the last few years help to put the drug's career into relation to other 'vegetable' narcotics, such as cannabis for example.[5]

It is necessary to point out that throughout history the term 'coca' has been accompanied by some ambiguity. In this book, coca refers to the South American plant cultivated for the native population as food substitute, relief against altitude sickness, and minor stimulant. For more than 150 years, coca has been known as the raw material to produce cocaine, which faced global restrictions

4 This argument has also been echoed by manufacturers of coca products today, for example by Coca Nasa who produces energy drinks and beer containing coca in Columbia. See Maria Luisa Paul and Bryan Pietsch, "Indigenous Colombian coca company challenges Coca-Cola's trademark," *The Washington Post*, 118th June 2025, https://www.washingtonpost.com/world/2024/09/15/coca-nasa-cola-columbia-indigenous/.

5 According to Victorians, 'vegetable' narcotics are drugs that are natural and unmanufactured. For example, coca leaves can be consumed as such by chewing or as tea, opium is dried poppy juice that has been freed from impurities and can be drunken or smoked, and cannabis is consumed crushed by eating or smoking. Other common 'vegetable' narcotics in British nineteenth century society included belladonna and henbane. See Mortdecai Cooke, *The Seven Sisters of Sleep* (London: James Blackwood, 1860) and "The Narcotics we indulge in," *Blackwood's Edinburgh Magazine* 74, no. 457 (November 1853), 605–28.

in the early twentieth century as the number of consumers for recreational purposes rose significantly which caused concerns for public health. It is crucial to point out that at no time should coca be seen synonymous with cocaine which seems to be a problem in twenty-first century rhetoric on the subject. Although they share the same botanical origins, the raw material and purified product are very different in their geographical, cultural, and historical backgrounds. As a result of these circumstances, expectations for the medicinal and recreational value of both substances have varied greatly and has also raised different responses. On few occasions, I look at similarities and differences wherefore the reader needs to pay close attention when I speak of coca or cocaine, or both, to avoid confusion or misinterpretation. Coca is also not to be mistaken with cocoa, which is the raw material for chocolate. Wherever quoted as 'cocoa' on the following pages, the error occurred in the original sources and is highlighted by underlining, bold font, or in a footnote.[6]

Whenever the term 'drug' is used, I refer to the definition as found in the Oxford Dictionary for Nursing: "any substance that affects the structure or functioning of a living organism."[7] This also concurs with the Victorian understanding of 'drugs.' Given this definition, the term 'drugs' does not have strictly negative connotations, and it cannot be compared to the use of the word in other languages, such as *Drogen* or *Betäubungsmittel* in German nowadays.[8] After all, the term has experienced various interpretations within different historical contexts which needs to be taken into consideration.

Within these pages, historical place names such as "Bombay" and "Ceylon" are used in alignment with the terminology found in published and unpublished sources of the nineteenth and early twentieth centuries. This reflects the historical context of the discussion while acknowledging that these names have since been changed to "Mumbai" and "Sri Lanka," respectively, following political and cultural shifts.

By narrowing down the broad history of narcotics to the history of coca in nineteenth-century Britain, the topic gains more depth of focus. Especially the

---

6 This resemblance to other words was already noted in Victorian times, "The History of Coca," *The Lancet* vol. 173 issue 4459 (13th February 1909), 485.

7 Elizabeth Martin and Tanya McFerran, *A Dictionary of Nursing* (Oxford: Oxford University Press, 2008), 144.

8 Betäubungsmittelgesetz – BtMG, §1, accessed 18th June 2025, https://www.gesetze-im-internet.de/btmg_1981/__1.html, Neue-psychoaktive-Stoffe-Gesetz (NpSG), §2, accessed 18th June 2025, https://www.gesetze-im-internet.de/npsg/__2.html.

botanical and economic contexts of the history of coca have often been overlooked by historians although they played an important role in the career of coca. [9] In this book, I take a closer look at interactions between actors that contributed significantly to the introduction of the drug, especially those that led to the creation of a closely tied network originating at Kew. Valuable sources in that respect that have yet been skipped by historians, but are part of this work, include Bills of Entry and personal communication between a variety of professions.

This internal framework was then complemented by external factors such as cultural attitudes and social currents which highlight interdependencies between the actors and circumstances constituting the surrounding conditions that shaped the career of coca in Britain. The history of coca in nineteenth-century Britain was shaped by mutual interactions and interdependencies between cultures, countries, developments, and people wherefore it is analysed here as an entangled history.[10] As a result, this book offers a more accurate understanding of this complex topic, provides new insights, and challenges the established narrative that coca played an insignificant role in the history of narcotics in Britain.[11]

---

9 Gootenberg mentioned the botanical context in passing in *Andean Cocaine*: […] European powers (Britain, the Netherlands, and to a lesser extent France and Germany) began working on formal coca colonization schemes – a "botanical imperialism" that would transplant coca from the Andes and befit their expanding tropical colonies," 30. Similarly, Steven B Karch summed up British cultivation efforts of coca in two paragraphs before dedicating a whole chapter to Dutch cultivation in Java in *A Brief History of Cocaine* (Boca Raton: CRC Press, 1998), 71–81.

10 See footnote 9, as well as Brian Inglis, *The Forbidden Game. A Social History of Drugs* (New York City: Charles Scribner's Sons, 1975), who – as the title indicates – took a social approach to the history of drugs just like Terry M Parssinen, *Secret Passions, Secret Remedies. Narcotic Drugs in British Society 1820 – 1930* (Philadelphia: Institute for the Study of Human Issues, Inc. 1983), who narrowed it down to Britain during roughly a century. A cultural viewpoint was then taken by B Milligan in *Pleasures and Pains: Opium and the Orient in Nineteenth-Century British Culture* (Charlottesville: University Press of Virginia, 1995), similar to the most recent work by Douglas Small, *Cocaine, Literature, and Culture, 1876–1930* (London: Bloomsbury, 2024), that also encompassed a literary outlook. A political history of opium can, for example, be found in Timothy Brook and Bob Tadashi Wakabayashi, eds., *Opium Regimes: China, Britain, and Japan, 1839–1952* (Berkeley: University of California Press, 2000).

11 Interdependencies have often been ignored in other histories of narcotics, for example in *Andean Cocaine: The Making of a Global Drug* (Chapel Hill: The University of North Carolina Press, 2008) where Paul Gootenberg primarily focuses on economic circum-

A network analysis initially developed by Jan Fuhse for cultural sciences thus provides a powerful tool to make the coca network visible and explain social circumstances that accompanied the introduction of coca as a novelty on the opium-sodden British market.[12] The Royal Botanical Gardens at Kew became the centre of this network that was constructed for and around coca. Institutional theory therefore explores how Kew was established and became accepted as an authoritative institution in the dissemination of coca knowledge.[13] It also shows Kew's integration into a wider nexus compromising medicinal, economic, and political aspects that shaped coca's career in Victorian Britain.

Fuhse's network analysis is then closely tied to Georg Simmel's theory of *Vergesellschaftung*, which medical historians Wolfgang Eckart and Robert Jütte used to better understand interrelations in medical history.[14] This theory helps to explain the relationships between actors involved with coca at Kew and how coca's mode of application and consumption changed when it was introduced to the British and European markets. Simmel also influenced the concept of "commodification," which is important because coca became a commodity in late nineteenth-century Britain through a network starting at Kew that quickly shifted and evolved towards economy and pharmacy.[15] At the same time, coca's

stances and implications of coca and cocaine trade. This is also evident in *From Silver to Cocaine: Latin American Commodity Chains and the Building of the World Economy, 1500–2000*, ed. Steven Topik, Carlos Marichal, and Frank Zephyr (North Carolina: Duke University Press, 2006). Whereas Berridge and Edwards take on a cultural approach in *Opium and the People*, they neglect economic, pharmaceutical, and political aspects.

12 Jan Fuhse, *Social Networks of Meaning and Communication*. (Oxford: Oxford University Press, 2022), 8.

13 For more on institutional theory see Lynne G Zucker, "The Role of Institutionalization in Cultural Persistence," *American Sociological Review* 42, no. 5 (1977), 726–43 and Christine Ahrend, Audrey Podann, and Johanna Schabert. "Institutionalisierung," in: Tobias Schmohl and Thorsten Philipp, eds., *Handbuch Transdisziplinäre Didaktik* (Bielefeld: transcript Verlag, 2021), 141–50.

14 *Vergesellschaftung* assumes that different spheres of reality exist independently of each other but that they only unfold their power through interdependence which constitutes a society that is connected through common interests, see Georg Simmel, *Soziologie. Untersuchungen über die Formen der Vergesellschaftung* (Leipzig: Duncker und Humblot, 1908), 6, 7; Wolfgang Uwe Eckart and Robert Jütte, *Medizingeschichte. Eine Einführung* (Köln: Böhlau Verlag, 2014), 176.

15 For an explanation of the term see: Albert Borgmann, "A Moral Conception of Commodification," in: Nico Stehr, Christoph Henning, Bernd Weiler, eds., *The moralization of the markets* (New York, London: Routledge, 2017), 194 and Lisa Erlenbusch, "Kommod-

rise as a commodity was linked to its *Politisierung* which posed the last stage in its career.[16] Although British politicians were primarily concerned with opium as their most important commodity in the empire, pressure from other countries about the new narcotic cocaine led Britain to rethink its position. This *Politisierung* resulted in legal restrictions on coca and cocaine, ending coca's time as an unrestricted drug.

I start this book by examining contrasting cultural attitudes towards coca through first-hand reports by Spanish, German, French, and Italian explorers to illustrate the role of coca as a cultural marker for the native populations in serving both as food and medicine.[17] Drawing on personal communication of British botanists across the globe with the Royal Botanical Gardens at Kew, I also explain cultivation efforts in the vast British Empire and the creation of a coca network. [18]

Chapter II then explores the economic aspects of the career on coca using British diplomatic and consular reports, as well as Bills of Entry of the ports in Britain to provide details about the cultivation, manufacture, and trade of coca.[19] I also take a closer look at the German-Peruvian, French-Peruvian, and British-South-Asian axes here.

---

ifizierung Und Ihre Grenzen. Betrachtungen zu Markt und Gerechtigkeit" (MA Thesis, Karl-Franzens-Universität, Graz, 2018), 11, 13. For a collection of essays on commodification see Sabine Coelsch-Foisner und Christopher Herzog, eds., *For Sale! Kommodifizierung in der Gegenwartskultur* (Heidelberg: Universitätsverlag Winter, 2021).

16 For a historical analysis of the term see Martin Rhonheimer, "Politisierung und Demokratiekritik: Anmerkungen Zur Geschichte des Politisierungsbegriffes," *Archiv Für Begriffsgeschichte* 29 (1985): 138–46.

17 Compare, for example, de Zárate and Nucio, *Historia del des cubrimiento y conquista del Peru*, H A Weddell, *Voyage Dans le Nord de la Bolivie et dans les Parties Voisines du Perou ou Visite au District Aurifère de Tipuani* (Paris: P. Bertrand, 1853), Paolo Mantegazza, *Quadri della natura umana. Feste ed ebbrezze. Volume II* (Milano: Giuseppe Bernardoni, 1871), and Eduard Poeppig, *Reise in Chile, Peru und auf dem Amazonenstrome, Während der Jahre 1827–1832* (Leipzig: Friedrich Fleischer, 1836).

18 Personal communication of this kind can be accessed at the Kew Royal Botanic Gardens Archive, London, UK.

19 See Diplomatic and Consular Reports on Trade and Finance of various countries between 1887 and 1911 on ProQuest. See Customs Bill of Entry for Liverpool between 1855–1899 and for London between 1880–1900 at the British Library, London, UK. Mislabelling of coca will also be addressed here. The Customs Bill of Entry hardly mentioned cocaine as a single-standing commodity since it was primarily compromised under "merchandize" or "drugs." However, given that British pharmaceutical companies started producing and selling cocaine products, the narcotic must have been imported

In the third chapter, I focus on the role of the pharmaceutical industry for the career of coca by analysing a variety of articles and reports by pharmaceutical and medical experts, as well as advertisement.[20] They explain the purification process of coca into cocaine and provide more information about coca research while also shedding a light on negative connotations that evolved at the end of the nineteenth century.

The following chapter deals with sociocultural influences on the trajectory of coca in nineteenth-century Britain, particularly the cultural dissimilation, by an examination of articles in newspapers and magazines. It demonstrates the public's reaction to those two new narcotics, highlights the challenges that came with their consumption, and compares these with Germany as the centre for cocaine research and production at the time. This chapter furthermore provides an analysis of the blurred line between medicinal and recreational consumption, primarily in fiction, where concerns surrounding morality, addiction, and crime posed a prelude to political restrictions on narcotics after the turn of the century.[21]

The last chapter thus analyses how both coca and cocaine went from medical marvel to political menace analysing parliamentary papers and letters between the British government and government officials.[22] They reveal how the

---

from either South American countries or Germany, where Merck was the primary producer, after the 1870s at the latest.

20 Compare Carl Koller, "On the Use of Cocaine for Producing Anaesthesia on the Eye," transl. J N Bloom, *The Lancet*, Vol. 124, Issue 3197 (6th December 1884), 990–92, George Mivart, "Cocaine," *British Medical Journal* (6th December 1884), 1131, or Ralph Stockman, "Reports to the Scientific Grants Committee of the British Medical Association. Report on the Coca Alkaloids," *British Medical Journal* (11th May 1889), 1043–1046. The Wellcome Institute in London, UK holds plenty of ephemera and recipe books from Allen & Hanbury's, as well as the archives of Merck in Darmstadt, Germany.

21 Compare J H Baldock, "The Abuse of Narcotics," *The Times*, 15th January 1880, Chas Bell Taylor, "The Dangers of Cocaine," *The Lancet*, Vol. 126, Issue 3249 (5th December 1885), 1070, or Kailas Chunder Bose, "Cocaine Intoxication and its Demoralizing Effects," *British Medical Journal* (26th April 1902), 1020–1022. For an example in fiction, see Arthur Conan Doyle, *The Sign of Four* (London: Spencer Blackett, 1890) and Arthur Conan Doyle, "Adventures of Sherlock Holmes. Adventure VI – The Man With the Twisted Lip," *The Strand Magazine* Vol. II (Jul-Dec 1891), 623–637.

22 Compare HC Deb and HL Deb between 1839 and 1912 on UK Parliament's Hansard website https://hansard.parliament.uk/. Personal communication of that kind can be accessed at The National Archives, London, UK.

situation of illicit narcotic consumption and trade evolved, how specific issues were addressed and resolved, and eventually, these sources help to explain global restrictions.

At the end of this book, readers will find a concept for the career of vegetable narcotics based on my empirical findings. This can help to explain how botanical, economic, pharmaceutical, sociocultural, and political circumstances shaped the career of a vegetable narcotic. Comparing and contrasting this concept to those of two historians who have also suggested concepts for the careers of narcotics – Max Seige in 1912 and Hans Derks in 2012 – this shows if the concept developed here can be extended to other narcotics in history and thus serve as a template for future research.[23]

As opium has long been the most important narcotic in the history of the British Empire, it has produced an abundance of literature and historiography on the topic from a variety of perspectives.[24] Other drugs, however, have been neglected. Among them, coca deserves special attention. Like opium, coca was an exotic substance, but its career in Britain followed a very different path.[25] This publication therefore treats coca as an exceptional drug in British history

---

23 Max Seige, "Klinische Erfahrungen mit Neuronal," *Deutsche medizinische Wochenschrift*, 38 (1912), 1828–30; Hans Derks, *History of the Opium Problem. The Assault on the East, ca. 1600 – 1950* (Leiden: Brill, 2012).

24 From the early until the mid-twentieth century, the history of opium in Britain hardly occupied the minds of historians. It experienced a renewed interest after the 1960s with several political interpretations, including Chang Hsin-Pao, *Commissioner Lin and the Opium War* (Cambridge: Harvard University Press,1964), Cheng U Wen, "Opium in the Straits Settlements, 1867–1910," *Journal of Southeast Asian History* 2, no. 1 (1961), 52–75, and Amalendu Guha "Imperialism of Opium: Its Ugly Face in Assam (1773–1921)," *Proceedings of the Indian History Congress* 37 (1976), 338–46. From 1980s to the 2000s, historians then took on a more social and cultural approach as in the previously mentioned Berridge and Edwards, *Opium and the People* and Booth, *Opium: A History*, but also in Parssinen, *Secret Passions, Secret Remedies* and Milligan, *Pleasures and Pains*.

25 For the role of coca in the acquisition of revenue for the Spaniards in the sixteenth century compare Augustin de Zárate and Martin Nucio, *Historia del des cubrimiento y conquista del Peru, con las cosas naturales que senaladamente alli se hallan, y los sucessos que ha audio* (Casa de Martin Nucio, 1555), Don Antonio Julian, *La Perla de la America, Provincia de Santa Maria, Reconocida, Observada, y Expuesta en Discursos Historicos* (Madrid: Printed for Don Antonio de Sancha,1787), and Pedro De Cieza de León, *Crónica del Perú: El Senorío de los Incas*, ed. Franklin Pease G. Y. (Caracas: Fundación Biblioteca Ayacucho, 2005). Also compare "Cocaine," *Chambers's Journal of Popular Literature, Science, and Art* 3, no. 114 (6th March 1886), 147: "Cocaine flashed like a meteor before the eyes of the medical world, but, unlike a meteor, its impressions have proved to be enduring."

that is much more than just the raw material for the more potent and globally disparaged cocaine. Although several published and unpublished sources cover the botanical, economic, and political aspects of the history of coca, they have so far not received the attention they deserve. This book aims to change that to position coca within the broader history of narcotics in Britain.

Chapter I: From Incan to Imperial Leaf

1. Botanical Origins

The history of coca and its botanical origins date back several millennia with the earliest evidence being found on ancient artefacts from around 5000 BC.[1] It is likely that early hunter-gatherers in South America experimented with coca and discovered its marvellous properties before it became the sacred plant of the Inca around the same time of the High Middle Ages in Europe. The Inca lived in today's Peru and parts of modern-day Ecuador, Bolivia, Chile, and Argentina between the 13th and 16th Century AD where *Erythroxylon Coca*, as it became known in science, was widely cultivated there. The climate in Peru and adjacent countries such as Bolivia was perfect for growing coca since it required a mean temperature of about 17 degrees Celsius and sufficient precipitation. The coca shrub yielded leaves about one and a half years after planting and could be harvested up to four times annually which was a relatively easy task. Initially, the marvellous properties of the leaves made them a popular ingredient in rituals and increased its popularity among the aristocracy in Incan times. Common people wanting to use coca had to request permission from higher officials since it was considered a sacred plant.[2] However, due to

1 Kennedy, *Coca Exotica*, 13.

2 Joseph Acosta, *The Naturall and Morall Historie of the East and West Indies*, trans. E. G. (London: Printed by Val: Sims for Edward Blount and William Aspley, 1604), 273; Ferdinando Gorges, *America Painted to Life. The True History of The Spaniards Proceedings in the Conquests of the Indians, and of their Civil Wars among themselves, from Columbus his first Discovery, to these Later Times* (London: Printed for Nath. Brook at the Angel in Cornhil, 1659), 8.

coca growing abundantly, the habit rapidly spread among the middle and lower classes of society and became a cultural marker for the Inca as a whole. [3]

The natives preferred the fresh leaves over stored ones since they had the greatest effect after consumption and tasted better. Unbeknownst to them, the alkaloid content decreased in due course and after about a year of storage the coca leaves would not produce any significant effects.[4] Incas preferred chewing coca leaves with a small amount of lime (*llipta*) which enhanced the flavour and increased the potency in comparison to drinking coca tea although it was a common method of consumption, nonetheless. Males usually started chewing coca in their teenage years since it symbolised progression from childhood to adulthood. [5] From that age on, Incas would carry with them a little pouch where they kept their coca and *llipta*, and they would rarely be seen without a little ball in their mouths formed from the two ingredients. This ball, called *aculio*, was kept in the mouth until the effect wore off which usually occurred after a few hours. [6] Initially, coca chewing helped the Andean population to cope with high altitudes and treat vertigo while also alleviating pain, especially in the oral cavities and in gastrointestinal ailments. It also prevented fatigue during hard labour and it was beneficial to endure longer periods without food and drink, for example during the revolutionary wars that took place in today's Argentina, Peru, Venezuela, and Colombia between 1810 and 1825.[7] Although coca leaves alleviate hunger and have been a daily drug for South American native populations, scientifically they cannot be considered food.

As a result, coca's effects on the human body and mind were too fascinating for medical professionals to be neglected or forgotten so that increased re-

---

3 "Some Popular Remedies," *Chambers's Journal of Popular Literature, Science and Arts* 12, no. 577 (19th January 1895), 44; Mariani, *Coca and its Therapeutic Applications*, 22; Kennedy, *Coca Exotica*, 15, 26, 27; Douglas H Boucher, "Cocaine and the Coca Plant," *BioScience* 41, no. 2 (1991), 72; Courtwright, *Forces of Habit*, 46.

4 Poeppig, *Reise in Chile, Peru und auf dem Amazonenstrome*, 213.

5 Mariani, *Coca and its Therapeutic Applications*, 24, 25.

6 Ibid., 23.

7 Hooker, *Companion to the Botanical Magazine; Being a Journal, Containing such Interesting Botanical Information, as does not Come Within the Prescribed Limits of the Magazine; With Occasional Figures*; 265; Franz J F Meyen, *Outlines of the geography of plants: with particular enquiries concerning the native country, the culture, and the uses of the principal cultivated plants on which the prosperity of nations is based* (London: Printed for the Ray Society, 1846), 364, 365; "The Coca Chewers of Peru," *The London Saturday Journal* 2, no. 47 (23rd November 1839), 327.

search on the plant eventually revealed its magnificent powers in the Victorian Era. But before coca could enter the European stage as an exotic narcotic that would compete with the omnipresence of opium, the drug had to face several challenges upon the arrival of the first Europeans in the sixteenth century. As it turned out, South America was not only literally but also metaphorically an ocean away from Europe.

Similar to religious men eradicating opium from medicine in Europe during the Middle Ages, the Catholic Church prohibited coca chewing in Peru upon arrival of the conquistadores since it was disparaged as an 'Indian vice.'[8] In a conference of South American bishops in Lima in 1569, it was even called "*Un delusion del demonio*."[9] Coca was a novelty for Iberians who first arrived in South America and because of this disparagement the Inca were forced to give up their habit for several years. This initial prohibition of coca reflected a mix of reflected prevailing hierarchical views and a lack of understanding of its cultural significance until the Spaniards experienced for themselves that it was indeed a native necessity that would benefit the Spanish cause. Realising that the natives were unable to work in the silver mines without their daily supply of coca, they eventually allowed the natives to continue the practice but not without raising up to ten per cent taxes on the product.[10] In his *Crónica Del Perú* from 1550, conquistador Pedro de Cieza de León stated: "[Los indios] dicen que sienten poco la hambre y que se hallan en gran vigor y fuerza."[11] This way, the conquistadores took advantage of the natives being addicted to the drug to exploit their country not only for valuable metals such as gold and silver but also for coca. Besides of perceiving coca as a cash crop, the Iberians were impressed by the miraculous properties of coca to sustain labour and contemplated coca as a drug for workers back at home since it seemed a "cheap substitute for coffee and tea."[12] As de León further explained, some Spanish traders became rich from trading with coca in the Indian market and it was generally believed that coca "nunca dejará de ser estimada."[13]

8 "Some Popular Remedies," 44.

9 Transl.: "a delusion of the devil," Mortimer, *History of Coca*, 108.

10 Clements Markham, *Travels in Peru and India* (London: John Murray, 1862), 236; Kennedy, *Coca Exotica*, 37. The former spoke of 5% excise in 1591, the latter of 10%.

11 de Cieza Leon, *Crónica del Perú*, 248; transl.: "They [the Indians, KE] say that they feel little hunger and that they possess great vigour and strength."

12 Bauer, "Travel Medicine, Coca and Cocaine," 5.

13 de Cieza de Leon, *Crónica del Perú*, 248; transl.: "will never cease to be valued."

Surprisingly, though, Iberians did not bring back coca leaves to Europe in significant amounts but they brought with them knowledge about the existence of the plant. In 1555, coca was first mentioned in a Spanish book on the discovery and conquest of Peru, but it would take another roughly fifty years until it first appeared in an English publication. These publications in England were chiefly translations of Portuguese, Spanish or French first-hand reports from missionaries or travellers. They highlighted the value of coca for the native population which "satisfieth both hunger and thirst" and "gives them great courage" but also emphasised its value as a commodity.[14] Coca was first listed as a drug in Pomet's *Compleat History of Druggs* where he compared coca in South America to betel in Asia and to tobacco in Europe.[15] Still, none of these books included a drawing of the plant or a detailed description of its appearance, so the look of the plant remained a mystery to anyone who lacked the opportunity to travel to South America before the Victorian Era.

Nevertheless, a recent and most interesting toxicological study of archaeological remains in Italy seeks to tell a different story of the arrival of coca in Europe as it claims that coca consumption had already existed on the continent in the seventeenth century. Analysing the brain tissue of nine human remains in a crypt adjacent to a hospital in Milan, Italy scientists did not only find traces of *Papaver somniferum* (poppy), but also of *cannabis* and *Erythroxylon* (coca).[16] Whereas the former had been part of pharmacopoeias since Antiquity, the latter two were not. The Italian researchers claim that the amount of *Erythroxylon* and its by-products found in the brain tissue indicated coca chewing in these individuals which could also have occurred "near the time of death" but

---

14 Antonie Galvano, *The Discoveries of the World from Their First Originall Unto the Yeere of Our Lord 1555*, trans. Richard Hakluyt (London: Impensis G. Bishop, 1601), 87; de Zárate and Nucio, *Historia del des cubrimiento y conquista del Peru*, 17; Acosta, *The Naturall and Morall Historie of the East and West Indies*, 185, 273.

15 Pomet, *A Compleat History of Druggs, Written in French by Monsieur Pomet, Chief Druggist to the present French King, to which is added what is further observable on the same Subject, from Mess. Lemery, and Tournefort, Divided into Three Classes, Vegetable, Animal and Mineral; With Their Use in Physick, Chymistry, Pharmacy, and Several Other Arts* (London: Printed for R Bonwicke, William Freeman, Timothy Goodwin et al., 1712), 95.

16 Gaia Giordano, Mirko Mattia, Lucie Biehler-Gomez, Michele Boracchi, Alessandro Porro, Francesco Sardanelli, Fabrizio Slavazzi, Paolo Maria Galimberti, Domenico Di Candia, Cristina Cattaneo, "Forensic toxicology backdates the use of coca plant (Erythroxylum spp.) in Europe to the early 1600s," *Journal of Archaeological Science*, Volume 170 (2024), 2.

was at least “representative of an acute intake” rather than regular and prolonged consumption.[17] They concluded that this circumstance, together with the plant not appearing in the hospital's pharmacopoeia indicated either recreational consumption of coca leaves or the patient consuming it shortly before their admittance to the hospital. Giordano et al. also added that Milan being under Spanish rule at the time facilitated the availability of coca in situ through “a direct connection between the maritime sales and the city of Milan.”[18]

Although this study has been unprecedented and seems to show remarkable results that could influence the history of coca in Europe, its findings need to be treated with caution. The scientists detected traces of *Erythroxylon* in only two out of nine samples and their anthropological origin, i.e., their population affinity, could not be determined, just like for most of the human remains.[19] One of these two samples belonged to a middle-aged man who suffered from syphilis. These circumstances point towards another explanation not offered by the researchers of this study. Given that “[...] the presence of cocaine and metabolites of coca leaves exclude the possibility of environmental exposure to the plant” and the unknown origin of the human remains, it is possible that the two individuals arrived in Milan from an overseas journey from South America.[20] This explanation is also supported by the fact that Spain maintained trade relations between Milan and South America and that coca leaves deteriorated quickly on the overseas journey. Even if sufficient coca leaves had arrived in Italy at that time that had not lost a significant portion of their potency, it is highly questionable whether a patient that ended in a hospital for “impoverished and disadvantaged individuals” could have obtained those.[21]

Moreover, the argument that the consumers of coca discovered in a Milanese crypt were not European is reinforced by the detection of syphilis in one of the two positive samples. The illness was allegedly brought to Europe by the Columbian Exchange in the late fifteenth and sixteenth century, in which Iberians played a crucial role.[22] Consequently, this indicates that the individual examined by the researchers was a tradesman or assistant thereof who was

17 Giordano et. al., “Forensic toxicology,” 10, 11.

18 Ibid., 10.

19 Ibid., 3.

20 Ibid., 8.

21 Ibid., 2.

22 Kerttu Majander, Saskia Pfrengle, Arthur Kocher, et al., “Ancient bacterial genomes reveal a high diversity of Treponema pallidum Strains in early Modern Europe,” *Current Biology* 30 (19) (2020), 3788.

probably consuming coca against sea sickness before syphilis broke out after his arrival – several weeks pass before first symptoms are noticed.

Whether the findings of this study are truthful, this can only be confirmed through future archaeological studies and the study of contemporary documents. It can be helpful to look at Bills of Entry for Italy or specific duchies, such as Milan, at the time to confirm the much earlier arrival of coca leaves in Europe. It is desirable that more research is done on this specific topic which might require the history of the arrival of coca in Europe to be rewritten.

But for now, let's have a look at European expeditions to South America in the nineteenth century. From 1809 to 1824, Peru fought for independence from Spain which prevented many Europeans from travelling to the country. This changed after the Peruvian victory and several journeys were undertaken to gather scientific knowledge about this still vastly unknown terrain. Three German botanists stood out here: Carl Friedrich von Martius travelled through Brazil from 1817 to 1820, Eduard Poeppig travelled through the Western part of the continent from 1827 to 1832, and Franz Julius Ferdinand Meyen explored Peru on his journey around the world from 1830 to 1832. A little later, Swiss botanist Johann Jakob von Tschudi travelled through Peru from 1838 to 1842. These times also coincided with the era of Romanticism that first and foremost permeated German society and emphasised freedom, the connectedness to nature, and *wanderlust*.

The first publication of coca and a coloured drawing thereof appeared in Hooker's *Companion to the Botanical Magazine* in 1835. It was a translation of Eduard Poeppig's experiences with coca that he described in *Reise in Chile, Peru und auf dem Amazonenstrome* and that was published in Germany in the same year. The problem with this was, though, that Poeppig painted a very dark picture of coca and its consumers which Hooker inevitably accepted since he lacked experience in situ. It was a highly biased and racially discriminating report that clearly illustrated a feeling of superiority and resembled opinions of the Anti-Opium society a few decades later.

Poeppig started off to explain that "[u]eberall haben rohe Völker, nicht zufrieden mit den einfacheren Reizen, es sich angelegen sein lassen künstliche zu erfinden [...]. Je tiefer ein Volk auf der Leiter der geistigen Fähigkeiten steht, um so größer sind die ihm angenehmen Reizmittel [...]."[23] In this way, he described coca as a strong cultural marker for the indigenous population which

23 Poeppig, *Reise in Chile, Peru und auf dem Amazonenstrome*, 210, transl. Hooker, *Companion to the Botanical Magazine*, 162: "Rude nations have ever sought for artificial excitements,

he compared to consumers of alcohol and opium who would still be better off since the effects would not last as long and the vice was possible to be abandoned.[24] He claimed that coca was a "nothwendiges Uebel in Peru," a necessary evil, not only for the sake of the native population but also for traders such as the conquistadores who amassed a fortune with it.[25] He was also convinced that the effects of coca were greatly exaggerated. In successive pages he repeatedly stated that reports about its effects were "irrig," erroneous, and in conjunction with personal experiments he arrived at the following conclusion:

> Was die ersten Beschreiber Perus von den angeblich magenstärkenden, nährenden und kräftigenden Eigenschaften der Coca schrieben, hat man gläubig wiederholt, ohne zu erwägen, dass in jenem dünnen, membranösen, ziemlich geruch- und geschmacklosen Blatte keiner von den Stoffen in grösserer Menge vorhanden sein konnte, denen man Nahrhaftigkeit im gewöhnlichen Sinne des Wortes zutrauen darf.[26]

Why is it then that travellers before and after him had a much more positive impression of coca? One of the reasons was explained by Poeppig himself who mentioned that he lacked chemicals to conduct more detailed experiments with the leaves.[27] It is furthermore questionable whether he masticated the leaves, with or without lime, or drank infusions, and in what amount, or if he refrained from consumption at all and relied solely on his observations of the locals. These observations, however, illustrated several contradictions, for example when he described coca's volatile effect due to minute amounts of active principle in a leaf but then said coca consumers were "[f]ür alle

---

and the lower do a people stand in the scale of intellectual ability, so much the more attractive to them is that means of exhilaration [...]."

24 Poeppig, *Reise in Chile, Peru und auf dem Amazonenstrome*, 211.

25 Ibid., 254, 256.

26 Ibid., 215, 257, transl.: "What the first reporters of Peru wrote about the apparently stomach-strengthening, nutritious, and invigorating properties of coca was naively repeated without considering that in such a thin, membranous, quite odourless and tasteless leaf none of these substances which we ascribe nutritiousness could exist."

27 His fellow German pharmacist Friedrich Gaedcke also assumed a lack of chemical equipment that might have prevented a different verdict, see Friedrich Gaedcke, *Ueber das Erythroxylin, dargestellt aus den Blättern des in Südamerika cultivirten Strauches Erythroxylon Coca Lam* (Berlin: W. Moeser & Kühn, 1854), 9.

ernstere Lebenszwecke unbrauchbar" and faced premature death.[28] Similarly, he claimed that coca consumption was restricted to Peru but later argued it was consumed in Columbia, Bolivia, and Brazil as well.[29] It is therefore not too far-fetched to conclude that Poeppig more than likely did not consume coca to experience the effects first-hand. In his observations of the indigenous population, he was blinded by a supremacist and racist attitude which painted every consumer of coca with the same brush, regardless of the modes and amounts of consumption.[30]

Although Joseph de Jussieu, a pharmacist and graduate in medicine, was the first to send samples of the coca plant back home to his cousin in France while he was travelling through Peru in the eighteenth century, these samples were limited. Therefore, it would take almost a century until a detailed description of the coca plant appeared in an English publication. It was Sir William Hooker, future director of the Royal Botanical Gardens at Kew, who first published a translated extract of eleven pages from Poeppig's *Reise in Chile* that included not only a description of its appearance and cultivation but also the first coloured drawing of the coca plant.[31] Nevertheless, it still took more than two decades until coca leaves arrived in Europe in such an amount that would enable further examination. The results of these studies then fostered the importation of bigger amounts of coca that caused chemists and pharmacists to experiment with the new drug and introduce their products into the market.

Hooker's translation at times tried to moderate Poeppig's racial tones, as can be seen in the translation of the very first quote cited earlier, and a fellow botanist making a remark on coca a year later also sought a more positive statement. Lindley gave credit to previous travellers who highlighted coca's "remarkable power in stimulating the nervous system" and in a comparison with opium came to the conclusion that the negative effects of coca chewing did not succeed those of opium consumption.[32] Even a fellow German of Poeppig,

---

28 Poeppig, *Reise in Chile, Peru und auf dem Amazonenstrome*, 211, 212, 213, transl.: "useless for all serious purposes in life."

29 Ibid., 252.

30 See also quote from footnote 87.

31 Hooker, *Companion to the Botanical Magazine*, 161–170, including supplement between pp. 160–161.

32 John Lindley, *Natural System of Botany; or, a Systematic View of the Organisation, Natural Affinities, and Geographical Distribution, of the whole Vegetable Kingdom; together with the Uses of the most Important Species in Medicine, the Arts, and Rural or Domestic Economy* (London: Longman, Rees, Orme, Brown, Green, and Longman, 1836), 123.

Ernst Freiherr von Briba, judged two decades later that he found his statements "etwas hart und streng, sowohl in Betreff der moralischen Seite, als auch der physischen Einwirkung" which portrayed coca in "schwarzen Farben."[33]

Poeppig's fellow Germans von Martius and Meyen also had a less dramatic impression of coca consumption in Peru. Both reported that the coca habit was comparable to the opium habit in Turkey and to tobacco consumption in other countries.[34] They noted that the habit was universal among the native population and needed to conduct their daily routines wherefore huge amounts were consumed. Judging from their report, von Martius was the one who also tried coca chewing himself and arrived at the conclusion that coca was a "Sorgenbrecher" but should not be consumed in excess or by neurasthenic people.[35] In any way, neither portrayed the coca habit in such a bad light as Poeppig did and they also refrained from ascribing it the same devastating effects as excessive opium consumption.

A similar sympathetic opinion of coca was held by von Tschudi who was the first to deliberate a possible trade of coca between Peru and Europe and discussed its benefits for Europeans. In a small but significant footnote, he explained that twenty-five pounds of coca cost an average of six Spanish dollars, which equalled to around 40 shillings or two British pounds, but that transport to the coast and across the ocean, together with import duties would greatly increase the price.[36] Twenty-five pounds lasted a moderate *coquero* about a year and would cost him nearly one shilling a week if consumed in Peru.[37] Taking into consideration the additional costs for shipping and duties and the average salary of a British labourer which ranged around 25 shillings a week and was

33 Ernst Freiherr von Briba, *Die Narkotischen Genußmittel und der Mensch* (Nürnberg: Wilhelm Schmid, 1855), 161; transl.: "a bit harsh, both in the moral aspect and its physical effects," "black colours."

34 C F P von Martius, *Reise in Brasilien auf Befehl Sr. Majestät Maximilian Joseph I. Königs von Baiern in den Jahren 1817 bis 1820 gemacht von weiland Dr. John. Bapt. Von Spix und Dr. Carl Friedr. Phil. von Martius, Dritter und letzter Theil* (München: Friedr. Fleischer, 1831), 1169; Meyen, *Outlines of the geography of plants*, 15.

35 Von Martius, *Reise in Brasilien*,1169; transl.: "worry breaker." Neurasthenic people were those who allegedly possessed weak nerves.

36 J J von Tschudi, *Travels in Peru, During the Years 1838–1842, on the Coast, in the Sierra, across the Cordilleras and the Andes, into the Primeval Forests*, trans. Thomasina Ross (London: David Bogue, 1847), 456; W G Sumner, "The Spanish Dollar and the Colonial Shilling," *The American Historical Review*, Vol. 3 No. 4 (Jul. 1898), 618.

37 Coca chewers reportedly consumed an average of 1–1.5 ounces of coca leaves a day which amounts to 365–547.5 ounces, or 22.8-34 lbs a year.

just enough to feed his family, chewing coca in Britain would have been a costly venture.[38] Nevertheless, von Tschudi was the first explorer in the early nineteenth century who contemplated coca's use for more than botanical purposes: He saw its potential as a commodity that could contribute to the economy along the South American-European axis.

Like Poeppig and Lindley, von Tschudi also made comparisons from coca to other drugs to make it relatable for foreigners. His observations were based on his own experience with chewing coca and drinking coca tea on his journeys through Peru and he found the plant to be highly nutritious, conducive to health, and preventative in altitude sickness.[39] He furthermore claimed that coca possessed similar narcotic powers like opium in producing "sensibility of the brain" and wearing out "mental vigour and activity," but that it did not cause "a total alienation of the mental powers or induce[d] sleep" as opium did.[40] Subsequently, he recommended coca for sailors to sustain hard labour on strenuous journeys and for the general public since it did not have the same injurious effects as liquor.[41]

What is striking about this period is that it was marked by an absence of British explorers who travelled to Peru and reported about the coca plant. This could have been one reason why the drug arrived significantly late in Britain as compared to countries on the continent. Charles Darwin, who travelled to and along the coast of South America on the *Beagle* in the 1830s, did not mention the plant in his reports which is surprising given the extent to which it was used among the native population.[42] The scarcity of other British explorers can be explained by the circumstance that romanticism with its *wanderlust* was primarily a German phenomenon and its impact in Britain was limited. Furthermore, a lack of funding might have prevented other British explorers to travel to Peru – the Royal Geographical Society, for example, had only been founded in 1830.[43]

38 Liza Picard, "The working classes and the poor," British Library, accessed 18th June 2025, http://www.bl.uk/victorian-britain/articles/the-working-classes-and-the-poor.

39 Von Tschudi, *Travels in Peru*, 452, 453, 454.

40 Ibid., 451, 452.

41 Ibid., 457.

42 Only in a later publication on native languages does he make a brief reference to coca chewing of the Inca in Peru.

43 Dane Kennedy, "British Exploration in the Nineteenth Century: A Historiographical Survey," *History Compass* 5/6 (2007), 1886.

In the 1850s, expeditions for scientific purposes experienced a renewed upturn and produced more detailed knowledge about the coca plant and its mode of action. Botanist and physician Hugh Algernon Weddell, who was born in Britain but grew up and lived in France, accompanied his colleague Adrien Henri de Jussieu on multiple journeys during which he made his first encounter with the coca plant. His reports were published in France and England, but it was Jussieu's uncle Joseph who had sent the first samples of the coca plant to Europe in 1749.[44] However, this delivery only served the expanding of botanical knowledge rather than initiating further inquiries into its possible contribution as a medicine.

Jussieu's colleague Weddell was aware of the controversial depictions of the coca habit and greatly opposed Poeppig's narrative. He highlighted coca as an important product of commerce for the Spanish during the time of the Iberian conquest and explained that it still made up around 10% of the internal revenue in Bolivia.[45] Judging from his own indulgence in coca tea, Weddell concluded that its effects differed from the actual coca chewing in only producing an "excitation légère" and occasional insomnia.[46] In reference to Poeppig, he assumed that he and others who compared the coca habit to the opium habit in its pernicious effects must have bestowed too much credibility in badly informed people and exaggerated their accounts, although he admitted that Europeans unaccustomed to the habit might in fact experience some sort of discomfort.[47] Weddell concluded from his self-experiments that coca cannot be compared to tea, coffee, or alcohol since its effects were slower and steadier and affected the nervous system as a whole.[48]

A few years later, the first British explorer in South America to report firsthand about the coca plant was Clements Markham. In *Travels in Peru and India*, he described the historical and sociocultural significance of coca leaves for the native population, requirements for its cultivation, and its medicinal value. Markham also explained the Spanish encounter with coca and how this affected the economy. For him, his own personal observation and frequent consumption of coca served as evidence which made him a sympathetic advocator of the leaf: "[...] [O]f all the narcotics used by man, coca is the least injurious,

44 Sigmund Freud, "Ueber Coca," *Centralblatt für die gesamte Therapie* 2 (1884), 293.

45 Weddell, *Voyage Dans le Nord de la Bolivie*, 249, 516.

46 Ibid., 528; transl.: "light excitement."

47 Ibid., 529.

48 Ibid., 532, 533.

and the most soothing and invigorating."[49] Nevertheless, he also relied heavily on reports by Poepping, von Tschudi, and Weddell. Markham was aware that his report was published comparatively late, as he referenced the discovery of cocaine in Germany a few years prior, and this is also the report's disadvantage: It was published at a time when it was obsolete as the information he provided had already been known for more than three decades.

2. Network Beginnings

The comparatively late British engagement in the coca trade in comparison to other European countries, such as France and Germany, raises questions as to its exceptionality in the history of narcotics. For almost a century, opium, not coca, was the dominant narcotic on the British market and crucial for its economy, particularly through the revenue gained from its trade in China. This commodity significantly contributed to the British economy, next to the revenue derived from cotton and tea, and helped maintain economic stability within the Empire.[50] As the Prime Minister said in 1880: "The Indian revenue never can be solid and substantial so long as it is largely dependent on the opium revenue."[51]

In contrast to opium, coca posed several challenges for the British Empire. It could not be as easily cultivated there as the plant required specific geographical and climatic conditions that initially could not be found within the imperial realm.[52] Consequently, the British faced difficulties in establishing a stable and profitable coca supply chain. These environmental limitations required the British to initiate botanical and cultivation trials across various regions of their Empire to reduce reliance on South American sources.[53] As trade

49 Markham, *Travels in Peru and India*, 238.

50 Booth, *Opium and the People*, 139, 140.

51 HC Deb 4th June 1880 col. 1228.

52 There are roughly 250 different species of coca of which three yield a significant amount of the alkaloid cocaine: *Erythroxylon coca*, *Erythroxylon novogranatense*, and a subspecies of the latter, *Erythroxylon truxillense*. Botanical trials, as explained in the following, revealed that coca does not necessarily require the altitudes of the Andes to be cultivated.

53 Compare "We Have More than once Called Attention," *The Times* (28th December 1889), 7: "For this purpose [to extract cocaine from coca leaves, KE] experimental cultivation

with coca-growing countries, such as Peru and Bolivia, also faced severe competition from other European nations, such as France and Germany, Britain thus wanted to become independent from the production and distribution of coca.[54] In combination with the environmental limitations, which required innovative cultivation efforts, this led to the creation of a coca network.

The imperial efforts to cultivate coca as well as the successive transatlantic coca trade required a well-thought-out network of specialists in various fields whose competencies intertwined and facilitated the introduction and success of the new drug on the British market. Investigating a variety of sources from the British Library, the Royal Botanical Gardens at Kew, the Wellcome Collection, and the National Archives, they show that coca was embedded in a nexus that in fact exceeded that of a trade network. It did not merely involve farmers, traders, and merchants, but also botanists, pharmacists, chemists, and physicians. Their personal and business communication reveal interdependencies and close ties that all served a primary goal: to make coca a colonial commodity.

To understand the layout of this network and how the ties between various actors were established and maintained, a network theory developed by Jan Fuhse constitutes a valuable tool. According to Fuhse, "social structures consist of expectations" that are shaped by the culture of the actors which facilitates opportunities and offers relationship models.[55] Culture is therefore located on a macro-level, individuals on a micro-level and social networks assume a place in the middle on a meso-level since they emerge from communication and meaning. The relationships in social networks then follow specific patterns and they carry meaning which are constantly renegotiated and vary in stability.[56] The meaningfulness of the coca network developed due to the increasing demand for the commodity the actors were dealing with and their ties to each other changed over time with the resurfacing of new information that guided the actors' expectations towards each other.

The initial stage of this network became evident in the communication for the exchange of scientific information, for example between Sir William Hooker, Dr Theodor Wilhelm Christian Martius, and Daniel Hanbury who also

has been undertaken [...] with results which are not unsatisfactory in themselves; but for commercial purposes South America holds the field [...]."

54 Gootenberg, *Andean Cocaine*, 26, 30.

55 Jan Fuhse, *Social Networks*, 7, 27.

56 Ibid., 27, 28, 33.

connected a close friendship. For twenty years between 1845 and 1865, Hooker had been the director of the Royal Botanical Gardens at Kew, Martius was a pharmacist, and his brother Carl Friedrich Philipp was a botanist, who travelled through north-eastern South America in the early nineteenth century.[57] Daniel Hanbury was a chemist who experimented with various substances to create medicine for the people. However, their interest in each other's disciplines facilitated the expansion of pharmacognosy, which the British Library explains "at that time meant a close study of [a drug's] botanical and geographical origins."[58]

Although this network sounded predestined for success concerning the introduction of coca, their communication was characterised by a surprising absence of it. Hanbury regularly wrote to both Martius and Hooker, but the content of the letters regarded other plants, such as Cinchona which was also produced in South America. This absence indicates that the knowledge about coca and its exceptional properties must have been limited to only a few people during the 1850s and 1860s which was when the three exchanged botanical and chemical information. As pointed out in a previous section, reports on coca only made it to Britain through translations of earlier reports by European explorers, so it is likely that Hooker, Martius, and Hanbury have come across an article or two on the plant but did not realise its potential for the European medicinal world. Contributing to that is also the fact that coca was still difficult to procure and very expensive, so even when cocaine was discovered in 1859, they did not expect widespread consumption in Britain. Unfortunately for them, neither Martius, Hooker, nor Hanbury lived long enough to witness the marvellous effect of subcutaneous administration of cocaine that would significantly increase the importance of coca in the medicinal world – they died in 1863, 1865, and 1875, respectively. Had they still been alive, this could have greatly accelerated the career of the drug in their home country, but instead, their descendants took on this challenging task.

Martius' nephew Carl Alexander took over the family's pharmacy in Erlangen, Germany and unlike his father and uncle witnessed the discovery of

---

57 "Martius Pharmacognostic Collection," Friedrich-Alexander Universität Nürnberg-Erlangen, accessed 18th June 2025, https://www.fau.eu/fau/history-and-remembrance/collections-and-museums/martius-pharmacognostic-collection/.

58 "Daniel Hanbury," British Museum, accessed 18th June 2025, https://www.britishmuseum.org/collection/term/BIOG229452.

cocaine. However, he did not follow their path but instead focussed on industrial chemistry, rather than botany and pharmaceutical chemistry. He would later become the founder of the Agfa company which specialised in aniline, a substance needed to produce dyes and other chemicals. Other family members carried on the work in the pharmacy that hosted an almost complete collection of natural raw materials used for the manufacture of drugs in the nineteenth century.[59]

Starting in the 1860s and reaching its peak in the 1880s, the actual coca network developed from the Royal Botanical Gardens at Kew. Fuhse argues that actors in a network do not necessarily have to be individuals but can also be corporate actors which is true for Kew at this particular time in history.[60] Although the directors assumed the most important role, there were also assistant directors and other employees responsible for personal communication which made sense given the amount of documents Kew received over the years. Consequently, Kew can be positioned in the centre of the network which enabled them to reach actors in the network on the periphery which were often linked to each other through business, friendship, or family ties.[61] It does not seem coincidental that the network's centre was both a dispensary of coca seeds and the centre for the collection of knowledge which made the reciprocal nature of relations within the network very obvious. Kew provided seeds and specimens to botanists in various parts of the Empire to initiate and encourage cultivation efforts, and it was an unwritten law that results thereof had to be reported back to the director to determine whether those had been successful or not.[62]

At Kew Gardens, Sir Joseph Dalton Hooker followed in his father's footsteps and became the director after his death in 1865. The earliest letter he received

---

59 Karl Knobloch, "Apotheker Ernst Wilhelm Martius und seine Söhne Carl Friedrich Philipp und Theodor Wilhelm Christian," Collegium Alexandrinum, Universität Erlangen-Nürnberg, last amended 5th December 2009, http://www.collegium-alexandrinum.de/martius-lebenslauf.html.

60 Fuhse, *Social Networks*, 52.

61 Compare, for example, the friendship between botanist and director at Kew William Hooker with pharmacist Wilhelm von Martius, as explained in the beginning of this chapter, the family ties between Wilhelm von Martius and his botanist brother Carl, or the business ties between chemist Daniel Hanbury and pharmacist William Allen who jointly founded pharmaceutical company Allen & Hanbury's.

62 There is no written evidence that seeds and specimens were sent from Kew in exchange for reports on their cultivation but experimental trials and reports thereof to superiors belonged to the tasks of a botanist.

on coca arrived in February 1867 from William Dixon living in Birmingham who expressed his happiness over obtaining coca seeds after "2 or 3 years' effort" from the Bishop of Huanaco "to whom [he was] indebted for these seeds indirectly."[63] He sent some of the seeds to Hooker hoping that he would be able to take better care of the cultivation since coca was "of far more value in a military point of view than Cinchona" and he also contemplated the possibility of cultivating it in Hindustan, India. About two years later, Dixon send some more coca seeds to Hooker reporting that they had "already germinated" and expecting that Hooker would be "as fortunate" with the ones enclosed.[64] However, the requests in these two letters were singular incidents during that time since it took almost two more decades until Hooker decided to seriously take on cultivation efforts in the Empire.

Only after cocaine became known as a valuable anaesthetic in Germany in 1884, Hooker and his successor Wiliam Thiselton-Dyer sent coca seeds and specimens to botanists in the Empire for cultivation trials and the responsibility rested with them to spread knowledge about successes thereof. The communication between the botanists and Kew came natural since most of them either worked for the gardens under colonial orders or had previously been associated with Kew in some way. In January 1885, W M Mitchell expressed his desire to introduce coca into Ceylon with the help of seeds provided by Kew and in February of the same year, J Cathcar White, a reporter from Edinburgh, made a similar request.[65] White also highlighted that cocaine was then sold at 2s 6d per grain which made him believe that "the process [of extracting it, KE] must be very costly indeed or the production very difficult."[66] A few months later, Frederick William Burbidge kindly asked where he could purchase coca seeds for the cultivation in India by relatives of a Reverend Dr Haughton.[67] All three mentioned challenges in procuring seeds, leaves, plants, or any informa-

63 William Dixon to Sir Joseph Dalton Hooker, 21st February 1867, Royal Botanical Gardens at Kew.

64 William Dixon to Sir Joseph Dalton Hooker, 24th February 1869, Royal Botanical Gardens at Kew.

65 M W Mitchell to Sir Joseph Dalton Hooker, 6th January 1885, Royal Botanical Gardens at Kew.

66 J Cathcar White to Sir Joseph Dalton Hooker, 17th February 1885, Royal Botanical Gardens at Kew.

67 Frederick William Burbidge to Sir Joseph Dalton Hooker, 30th October 1885, Royal Botanical Gardens at Kew.

tion about the purification process wherefore they thought it best to contact the director at Kew.

In Kew many threads surrounding the cultivation, purification, and medicinal value of coca ran together. Not only was it the centre from where seeds were sent into the whole world, but it was also the place where knowledge about coca was accumulated. The variety of correspondents with Kew show that besides of botanists, chemists, wholesalers, even reporters commenced communication with the director to obtain more information about the drug that had sparked so much curiosity on the European mainland. In February 1885, for example, Thomas Christy offered to support Kew in determining the cocaine content of leaves grown in Madras by Dr Bidie.[68] In May, the Montserrat Company Ltd under leadership of Joseph Sturge obtained six coca plants which he planned to ship to the eponymous island of Montserrat in the West Indies with the next steamer.[69] The plants were on their way mid-June and were marked as "goods," which supports the theory that coca was often not labelled as such during shipments.[70]

The first pharmaceutical chemist in general to publish a report on coca alone was William Martindale. He wrote to Thiselton-Dyer, who followed as director of Kew after Sir Joseph D Hooker, on 5th January 1886: "Sir[,] I intend publishing some notes on the Coca Plant (Erythroxylon Coca) and should be glad if you could spare me a sprig in flower of the plant from which to make a sketch or to make a lithographic illustration for my little monograph. If not in flower now, is there any probability of a plant bearing flowers shortly?"[71] His request must have been met with agreement since he wrote again ten days later to inform the director about his visit the following day during which an employee would show him the coca plants and "do [him] a Water Colour of the Coca Plant – from life in the Kew Gardens, just for any purpose."[72] Similar like many other pharmacists and chemists, Martindale did not have

68 Thomas Christy to Sir William Thiselton-Dyer, 2nd February 1885, Royal Botanical Gardens at Kew.

69 Joseph Sturge to Sir William Thiselton-Dyer, 30th May 1885, Royal Botanical Gardens at Kew.

70 Joseph Sturge to Sir William Thiselton-Dyer, 11th and 13th June 1885, Royal Botanical Gardens at Kew. See chapter II for more information on mislabelled shipments.

71 William Martindale to Sir Thiselton-Dyer, 5th January 1886, Royal Botanical Gardens at Kew.

72 William Martindale to Sir Thiselton-Dyer, 15th January 1886, Royal Botanical Gardens at Kew; underlining in the original.

the opportunity to travel to South America to witness the cultivation of coca by first-hand experience, but at least he managed to see it in person in his home country. Apparently, Martindale sought to provide the full picture in his monograph rather than merely the leaves which he could have obtained from wholesalers.

In November 1886, coca leaves were sent back to Kew for further chemical experiments regarding their alkaloid content for the first time. It was a small tin that arrived from Balaclava, Jamaica and E Bapeltvuy hoped to make it a "profitable industry" on the island if they yielded enough cocaine.[73] This notion was small but significant as for the first time, a botanist contemplated the cultivation of a plant for economic purposes in his region, rather than for the gathering of botanical knowledge alone. Bapeltvuy realised the potential of coca for the British market and sought support from Kew to seize this opportunity. He received an answer from Kew a month later but unfortunately, the content of the letter is unknown. It is likely, though, that the alkaloid content was too low to promise successful full-scale cultivation in Jamaica, as later sources confirmed.[74]

Individuals who did not work for Kew or in the field of botany also wanted to contribute to the research of coca and sent back seeds to Kew from various locations. In December 1886, C G Oliver-Jones offered Kew some seeds he "received from Peru" which were gladly accepted, although botanists doubted its "germinating powers" due to unknown circumstances of their delivery.[75] Eight weeks later, businessman Marlborough Robert Pryor similarly enclosed some coca seeds to his letter "on the chance of them being of some use."[76]

Judging by little communication about coca at Kew after 1886 until late 1888, botanists across the globe were seemingly busy with cultivation trials as the plant needed at least one and a half years to yield results.[77] The collections

---

73 E Bapeltvuy to Sir Daniel Morris, 25th October 1886, Royal Botanical Gardens at Kew; sender could not be clearly identified.

74 Coca leaves and their alkaloid contents, folios 25 and 26; W B Sapent, "Erythroxylon Coca," 6th February 1888, Royal Botanical Gardens at Kew; W B Sapent "E. Coca var. novogranatense," 6th February 1888, Royal Botanical Gardens at Kew; the coca leaves grown in Jamaica yielded 0.24% and 0.33% of crystallisable alkaloids, respectively.

75 C G Oliver-Jones to the Royal Botanical Gardens at Kew, 14th December 1886, Royal Botanical Gardens at Kew.

76 Marlborough Robert Pryor to Sir Thiselton-Dyer, 22nd February 1887, Royal Botanical Gardens at Kew.

77 Mariani, *Coca and its Therapeutic Applications*, 16.

at Kew accessible today hold specimens of coca leaves from St Lucia, Jamaica, Demerara, Java, Ceylon, Bengal, and India that were glued into a notebook and show that the ones grown in Demerara were by far the biggest whereas those grow on Caribbean islands were comparatively small.[78] With coca shrubs growing well in some areas of the British Empire, the Royal Botanical Gardens became more interested in the alkaloid content in the leaves which were tested upon their arrival back in London by Howard & Sons. Nevertheless, size did not predict the alkaloid content as the biggest ones yielded a meagre 0,22 to 0,34%.[79] The coca grown in different parts of India, especially in Ceylon, yielded the highest cocaine content with up to 0,60%. This was similar to the alkaloid percentage in leaves from Kew which amounted to 0,55% but unlike in India, they did not grow to a significant extent there.[80] The collection at Kew reveals that there had been several efforts to cultivate coca in different parts of the British Empire to discover a location where the plant grew abundantly and yielded a high alkaloid content. Determining these two prerequisites was the first step for British botanists before commencing cultivation on a bigger scale.

Out of all the cultivation efforts, the collaboration triangle between Kew, Howard & Sons, and William Burck in Buitenzorg, Java seemed very promising. In February 1888, Howard's company tested almost two dozen coca leaves samples from the West Indies and the East Indies that were provided by Kew.[81] The percentage of crystallisable alkaloids in the leaves ranged between zero and 0.6% with the leaves grown in India again yielding the most, as their analysis in the previous month had shown. It is very likely that the ones containing hardly any or no alkaloid lost their potency during transport due inappropriate storage and packaging. Burck's samples that he sent to Kew in late February and April were also forwarded to Howard for analysis, and since he knew that the best way to handle coca leaves was to treat them delicately like tea, it is probable

78 These "experimental cultivation" areas were also mentioned in "We Have More than once Called Attention," *The Times* (28th December 1889), 7.

79 Coca leaves and their alkaloid contents, folios 15, 16, 18, 21, 25, 26, 29, 33, Royal Botanical Gardens at Kew.

80 Alfred G Howard to the Director at Kew, "Analysis of Coca Leaves from Kew," 2nd January 1888.

81 Alfred G Howard to the Royal Botanical Gardens at Kew, "Specimens of Coca Leaves Sent from Kew," 9th February 1888.

that their alkaloid content was still determinable after their six-week journey from Burck via Kew to Howard.[82]

Burck's report on his experiments and experience with coca on Java is the most extensive one in the collection at Kew, although it compromises less than four handwritten pages. Nevertheless, his writings reveal a few interesting observations about the rising popularity of coca, the existence of different species, and references to other actors in the research on coca. Burck observed that "E. [*Erythroxylon*, KE] Coca has obtained a certain reputation on account of the alcaloïd" which "got lately such an important therapeutic significance."[83] He took this as an opportunity to cultivate the plant on Java where professor of chemistry and pharmacology Dr J F Eykman conducted an analysis of the leaves. According to him, the cocaine content – not general alkaloid content – amounted to 0.976% which is much higher than even crystallisable and uncrystallisable alkaloids combined in other specimens tested by Howard. Even with modern technology the best variety of *Erythroxylon* today yields a maximum of 0.96% of cocaine.[84] Given Eykman's professional background, Burck had little to doubt in his results but something must have gone wrong in the process.

As a consequence, Burck pondered upon the huge difference between the leaves from plants grown on Java and those grown in British India, particularly in Perideniya, Ceylon, although every botanist raised them from seeds obtained from T Christy & Co.[85] Instead of questioning Eykman's method of analysis, he suggested that the price of coca sold on the market should depend on the alkaloid content and went so far as "to warn against the purchase of seeds from elsewhere" which would obviously give him the most advantageous position in the cultivation and trade.[86] Yet at the same time, he quoted the director of the Colonial Museum in Haarlem, Amsterdam who said that the alkaloid percentage is usually not mentioned during sale on the English market even though much of the coca sold there was of "bad quality."[87]

---

82 William Burck to Daniel Morris, 10th April 1888, Royal Botanical Gardens at Kew.

83 William Burck, "Coca.," 6th September 1888, Royal Botanical Gardens at Kew.

84 T Plowman and L Rivier, "Cocaine and Cinnamoylcocaine content of thirty-one species of Erythroxylum (Erythroxylaceae)," *Annals of Botany* (1983), 645.

85 Burck, "Coca."

86 Ibid.

87 Ibid.

After 1886, Burgoyne, Burbidges, Cyriax & Farries became the primary address for Kew to determine the value of different varieties of coca. Frederick William Burbidge was a botanist at Kew and manufacturing chemist, as well as his brother Thomas Burbidge.[88] Together with chemist Thomas Farries, merchant Julius Cyriax, and wine merchant Peter Bond Burgoyne they owned a successful wholesale and export druggist business. When Kew sent them some coca leaves upon request, they were found to be "not the sort usually sold in the market" wherefore they were only worth 6d in contrast to the best quality sold at 1s 6d per pound.[89]

Two years later, the connection between Kew and the company became even more important as the seeds sown at botanical outposts now produced plants and the value of the leaves for the market had to be determined. It was still challenging for the wholesale druggist company to give Kew more information due to "an absence of demand here [i.e., Britain, KE]."[90] Henry Ramold, who corresponded with Kew on behalf of the company, estimated the value at 6d to 8d at the beginning of 1888 which he corrected to 10d to 1s 6d per pound at the end of the year.[91] He admitted that "very few parcels of Coca leaves now come before us on the market" and that there was "an absence of statistics of stocks here [i.e., Britain, KE]" which complicated a more precise valuation.[92] This is in accordance with ambiguous declarations of coca in the Bills of Entry as will be explained later. Ramold's statement holds even more weight since his employer was one of the biggest whole-sale and export druggist companies in Britain which had an extensive overview of the kind of drugs sold on the market. If even they did not come across regular or increasing coca shipments despite their scale of operations, there was either no mentionable business or a significant lack of customs declaration. I discuss

88 "Burbidge, Frederick William Thomas (1847–1905)," Natural History Museum on JSTOR, accessed 18th June 2025, https://plants.jstor.org/stable/10.5555/al.ap.person.bm000150594; "Burbidges and Company Limited Burgoyne," Science Museum Group, accessed 18th June 2025, https://collection.sciencemuseumgroup.org.uk/people/cp111975/burgoyne-burbidges-and-company-limited.

89 Thomas Farries to John Reader Jackson, 25th December 1886, Royal Botanical Gardens at Kew.

90 Henry Ramold to Kew Gardens, 25th January 1888.

91 Henry Ramold to Kew Gardens, 25th January 1888; Henry Ramold to Kew Gardens, 9th November 1888.

92 Henry Ramold to Kew Gardens, 9th November 1888.

both possibilities in the chapter on trade which points towards a combination of the two.

When it came to the purified product, there was yet a third possibility that Ramold brought up in his correspondence with Kew. He believed that "manufacturers of Cocaine [...] possibly [bought] the crude extract" directly from Peru which he had confirmed by American friends.[93] Ramold furthermore stated that "[s]ince the large quantities of Crude Cocaine arrived from Lima on the European markets, there has not been such an active enquiry & the price [of coca leaves, KE] has declined [...]."[94] These claims were backed up by British consuls in Peru who mentioned almost two dozen manufacturing posts of cocaine in the country in 1902.[95] Although there probably were not as many roughly 25 years earlier, Ramold rose awareness that the trade in coca leaves might not be as profitable as Kew had hoped for due to an increasing interest in importing the purified product to Europe.

At the end of the nineteenth century, the coca network originating at Kew had grown significantly and was branching out in various directions. It was particularly well-connected with professionals from different fields within the imperial realm and facilitated connections between them to further knowledge about coca. Enabling a constant flow of information and resources between these actors, Kew viewed itself as essential to the functioning of the network and it could be understood as the centre of the coca network in Britain.

Assuming this key role, the directors in Kew tried to gather as many sources on the topic as possible. In March 1889, they showed strong interest in new publications on coca and its alkaloids from Trinidad after hearing that the Government Analyst of Trinidad planned on publishing a report on the matter in the same year.[96] A letter was sent via the Secretary of State for the Colonies to request further information which was approved a few days later and then forwarded to the Colonial Office in the Caribbean where John McCarthy conducted his experiments.[97] Unfortunately, it took almost a year for Kew to hear back since the correspondence was overshadowed by McCarthy's unexpected

---

93 Ibid.

94 Henry Ramold to Kew Gardens, 5th December 1888.

95 Henry Ramold to Kew Gardens, 25th January 1888; Henry Ramold to Kew Gardens, 9th November 1888.

96 R G K to Edward Wingfield, 26th March 1889.

97 Edward Wingfield to Sir Thiselton-Dyer, 29th March 1889, Royal Botanical Gardens at Kew.

death. The governor of Trinidad, William Robinson, informed Colonial Secretary Baron Knutsford in London about the unfortunate news and that with his death "all enquiries ceased, and as his notes recording the result of his experiments cannot be found much valuable information has [he feared] been lost."[98] Nevertheless, he enclosed minutes of McCarthy which he thought might be of use for the director at Kew.

Government analyst McCarthy's minutes from June 1889 contained little promising results. He explained that there had been a committee appointed for the purpose on conducting experiments on *Erythroxylon Coca* to determine its medicinal value but that he had been the only one carrying them out. McCarthy could not ask the committee's other members "who neither witnessed the Experiments nor apparently evinced any interest in them" to sign their outcomes.[99] In addition, he remarked that he did not have sufficient time to conduct experiments on his own "with that rapidity which seems to be desired" and that it might be best to leave judgment on the medicinal value of coca up "to the Doctors."[100] It becomes clear that at least on Trinidad but possibly on other islands of the West Indies, too, there seemed to have existed a lack of interest in coca and its cultivation, much in contrast to the interest of the home country. McCarthy provided evidence for that in stating that committee members on the one hand, did not support him in experiments and on the other hand, did not seem to be interest in the matter at all. As a result, the committee had failed their mission, and it ceased with McCarthy's death.

Still, according to McCarthy's minutes, the British Foreign Office desired quick results which strongly points towards Britain being under pressure to gather more information on coca in order to become more competitive: "I cannot do it [the experiments revealing more about the medicinal value of coca, KE] with that rapidity which seems to be desired [by the Colonial Secretary, KE]."[101] Given that the letters between him and Kew had to be processed via the Secretary of the Colonies in London, it seems as if this attitude proceeded from the latter. This meant that the focus shifted from a solely botanical interest in

98 William Robinson to the Colonial Secretary Baron Knutsford, 1st February 1890, Royal Botanical Gardens at Kew; brackets in the original.

99 John McCarthy to the Colonial Secretary Baron Knutsford, 14th June 1889, Royal Botanical Gardens at Kew.

100 McCarthy to Baron Knutsford, 14th June 1889.

101 Ibid.

the plant towards an economic interest in coca which were both characterised by colonial motifs. Watching Germany and France becoming major players in the coca trade, Britain had to develop strategies to keep up pace with other European powers in acquiring a colonial commodity that had previously been in the hands of the Spanish.

Kew did not solely act as the primary actor responsible for coca but also made referrals where they thought fit. Ernst Louis Armbrecht, for example, who was specialised in homeopathy as a pharmaceutical chemist, wrote to the curator at Kew to purchase a coca plant from them in September 1886. Unable to fulfil the request, he was redirected to Christy & Co who should be able to help him in the matter.[102] This circumstance is what Fuhse calls "switchings," after Harrison White.[103] A switching occurs when an actor mentions a tie to another actor in his communication which results in changes in the network since it highlights the relevance of this particular tie.[104] It is not known if Armbrecht pursued the referral but it took him almost three years to send another letter to Kew to request for "engravings or lithographs" of coca which he emphasised was a request directed by the Secretary of the British Museum's directions for which he was "ready at once to forward the necessary fees."[105] In mentioning the Secretary of the British Museum, his request certainly carried more weight than his previous one but it is unknown whether Kew accepted it or redirected him again.

The decision to establish new reciprocal ties highly depended on the benefits Kew expected out of them. Private requests to Kew were rare incidents and usually remained unanswered, for example when a Mr S [?]urtin wrote in May 1886 if the climate of Florida would be suitable to grow coca there since he had two sons who could undertake the venture.[106] An employee just noted a short "and?" on the letter which indicates that the letter was put ad acta without any reaction on behalf of Kew. A month later, John C Collins from Gloucestershire first turned to Martindale for advice who directed him to Kew for the procurement of seeds to see if they grew in Assam, India.[107] In this case, Kew advised

102 Ernst Louis Armbrecht to the curator at Kew, 6th September 1886, Royal Botanical Gardens at Kew.

103 Fuhse, *Social Networks*, 50.

104 Ibid., 49, 50.

105 Ernst Louis Armbrecht to Kew, 16th August 1889, Royal Botanical Gardens at Kew.

106 S [?]urtin to Sir Thiselton-Dyer, 10th May 1886, Royal Botanical Gardens at Kew.

107 John C Collins to Sir Thiselton-Dyer, 30th June 1886, Royal Botanical Gardens at Kew.

him to turn to the botanical gardens in Madras or Ceylon. In July of the same year, Reverend Richard Baxendale of Maidstone also requested information to obtain seeds so that his son, who would set sail soon, could try growing them in Australia.[108] Although the letter showed a little note that it had been answered, it is unclear in what way. E S Gunn, who was the founder of the Metropolitan School of Pitman's Shorthand and who also had connections to Australia, similarly received a reply with suggestions on further readings on coca and the procurement thereof.[109]

Kew's position in the network was thus characterised by a selectivity that would ensure its centrality as the career of coca progressed. It is obvious that [?]urtin, Collins, Baxendale, and other private businessmen realised Kew's position at the centre of the coca network wherefore they tried their luck in obtaining seeds for cultivation purposes, albeit unsuccessfully. Judging from Kew's reactions to those letters, it furthermore becomes clear that trials for cultivation of coca within the British Empire were supported whereas those outside of it – in Florida – were not. Not only does this show that Kew rejected new relations in the network that seemed unprofitable for them, but it also contributes to the theory that Britain wanted to become an independent producer of coca without any involvement of other countries. This does not come as a surprise as it reduced competition with other countries and gave Britain the control over the supply chain of coca.

The evolution of the coca network then raises the question whether there existed a kind of master plan from the very beginning in which Kew took on the role of a patron that initiated network connections. Fuhse understands patronage as a link between "actors in an unequal exchange of services, support, and loyalty" which contributes to the patrons becoming "more powerful and more attractive with the number of clients."[110] It is questionable whether Fuhse's relationship frame of patronage can be applied to Kew due to its position at the centre of the coca network and the constant exchange of goods and information. Initially, the network started off as a friendship between botanists William Hooker, chemist Daniel Hanbury, and pharmacist Theodor W C Martius. This relationship contradicted that of a patronage and an unequal exchange was non-existent. However, those friendship ties disappeared after their deaths and ties had to be re-established when the network

108 Richard Baxendale to Sir Thiselton-Dyer, 19th July 1886, Royal Botanical Gardens at Kew.

109 E S Gunn to Sir Thiselton-Dyer, 13th August 1886, Royal Botanical Gardens at Kew.

110 Fuhse, *Social Networks*, 57.

expanded. During the 1880s, the relationship between Kew and botanists in the Empire was clearly defined as employer and employees in which the former provided seeds and specimens for the latter to plant who would than inform about the outcomes. These outcomes – or rather the information about the botanical properties – were then shared with chemists and pharmacists who would determine alkaloid content in exchange. Kew could then share this knowledge with wholesalers who equally shared their knowledge about market value and buying behaviours of consumers. In the case of successful cultivation, it was an economic win-win situation for both. For obvious reasons, these ties were not based on an unequal exchange of some sort, but reciprocal, and therefore do not fall under the 'patronage' framework.

Nevertheless, there is one relationship that has not yet been examined: that between Kew and private businessmen. Whereas they played a neglectable role in comparison to other ties – given the few instances of personal communication – their ties looked different to that of other professions. People such as Collins or Baxendale sought to enter the coca network in establishing ties to the central actor in the coca network, Kew Gardens. Trying to establish ties to the most popular actor(s) is what Fuhse calls "preferential attachment" but in this case it did not work out.[111] As private individuals, they did not have anything to offer in return such as chemical, pharmaceutical, or wholesale knowledge which could make for an equal exchange of service. Kew realised this and therefore refrained from creating stable ties with them within the network.

The strongest or most stable tie in the coca network was without doubt the one evolving from the initial friendship triangle between Hooker, Martius, and Hanbury. After Hanbury's death, his descendants continued his work at Allen & Hanbury's in developing and manufacturing drugs for the British market and it is likely that communication with Kew persisted. By 1908, the company whose products were often marketed as 'Allenbury's' sold six different kinds of medicine containing coca, including fluid extract, throat pastilles, medicated pastilles, compressed tablets, and wine with and without quinine.[112] This success must have been the result of continuous exchange of botanical and

111 Ibid.

112 *General List of Drugs, Pharmaceuticals, and the "Allenburys" Specialities* (London: Allen & Hanburys Ltd., 1908), 92, 111, 112, 138, 139,165, 210, 211, 224, 240; several additional drugs marketed by Allenbury's contained cocaine but this will be explained in a later chapter.

pharmacogenetic knowledge between Kew on the one side and pharmaceutical chemists on the other.

All in all, Kew's position within the coca network can be best described by that of a "bridging leader" since it had "a high number of affiliations in multiple sectors."[113] Fuhse distinguishes between this and three other types of leaders that are often labelled 'brokers' by other sociologists.[114] As a bridging leader, Kew was not only expert in what Fuhse terms "discursive positioning" but it was also a facilitator of new ties through aforementioned switchings.[115] This gave the institution a privileged position through the accumulation of knowledge about coca from the cultivation to the value on the market. Kew distributed seeds to various botanists in the Empire and functioned as a hub to exchange information about cultivation successes, chemical qualities, and possible medicinal benefits. In doing so, Kew established valuable and meaningful connections between botanists, traders, pharmacists, and businessmen who shared the common goal to make coca a profitable commodity on the British market. Referencing and recommending suitable contacts, the institution created opportunities for collaborations between specific professions that yielded tangible benefits for the coca trade.

The network furthermore proved that it was adaptable and innovative in reacting to changes, for example when some regions did not provide satisfactory results in the cultivation of coca or when the amount of alkaloid in the leaves required pharmaceutical analysis and assessment that Kew could not conduct themselves. Another example was the transport of the plant: realising that whole coca plants would rot on their overseas journey, and that coca leaves would lose their potency, Kew decided to send seeds in sealed tin boxes instead. This improved positive feedback from botanists in British territories overseas and fostered cultivation efforts.

Kew's success in establishing a coca network was not only determined by the quality of its connections, but also by the quality of its content. Research conducted by botanists throughout the British Empire became relevant to more than just the Botanical Institute in the motherland, as it provided valuable data for pharmacists and wholesalers who in turn provided Kew with the data they gathered themselves. This meant that communication between the

113 Fuhse, *Social Networks*, 67.

114 See, for example, Martijn Koster and Yves van Leynseele, "Brokers as Assemblers: Studying Development Through the Lens of Brokerage," *Ethnos* 83 (5) (2018): 803–13.

115 Fuhse, *Social Networks*, 67.

actors in the network – primarily facilitated by Kew as the nodal point of the network – was regular and worked efficiently.

Over the course of more than five decades, the coca network originating at Kew grew consistently due to its adaptability, quality of connections, and quality of content. Carefully choosing new actors for its network, it ensured that they contributed to its goal to make coca a commodity that had a British supply chain independent from other South American or European countries. Although that goal was not yet clear when Hooker, Martius, and Hanbury exchanged friendly letters, it became more concrete with the advanced knowledge about coca's properties. It is noteworthy that despite the rather insignificant amount of the plant cultivated in India, as compared to South American countries, and its poorer quality which required a different method of extraction for the alkaloid, Indian-grown coca was also used for the pharmaceutical industry in Britain.[116] Consequently, Kew was in the driving seat to determine the future of coca in Britain.

The network surrounding Kew put an emphasis on the botanical aspect of coca but also established ties to other disciplines which constituted the first phase in the career cycle of the drug in Britain. Botanists laid the groundwork and significantly contributed to the expansion of a coca network, but foci shifted in successive decades. It was only natural that once the circumstances of mass cultivation, location, and organisation thereof were set that other actors gained in importance. Whereas the time up to the early 1880s was characterised by a highly active botanical centre at Kew, both economic aspects and the pharmaceutical industry became more relevant in the mid- to late-1880s. This was accompanied by medicinal developments which caused all three disciplines to be intertwined and develop in dependency of each other. As a result, Kew's role in the coca network gradually diminished but its role in initiating the network in the first place was crucial, nonetheless.

116 Compare footnotes138 and 139. For a more detailed examination of coca's role regarding the British pharmaceutical industry, see chapter III. When it came to the plant's alkaloid, British government officials reported that "the present demand and price of the drug d[id] not suffice to make the production of cocaine [in India, KE] pay," House of Commons, *Statement exhibiting the Moral and Material Progress and Condition of India during the Year 1890–91* (London: Eyre and Spottiswoode, 1892), 151.

Chapter II: The Transatlantic Coca Trade

1. Prelude

For the career of coca from the sixteenth until the mid-nineteenth century, coca's ability to sustain labour was the primary reason that made the conquistadores change their minds on the drug. They realised that it could contribute to their revenue in introducing duties and taxes on the leaf and they often used it instead of money to pay mine workers which saved them a lot in expenditure and contributed to an increase in wealth. Some Spaniards even became coca traders in Peru because it was a lucrative business and it certainly added to the Catholic Church's shift of opinion.[1] Unsurprisingly for a colonial power, the Spanish thought bigger in shipping coca leaves back to Europe but transportation was still too underdeveloped for such a venture: "[Coca] puderia ser un ramo de comercio ventajosisimo para España, salud de la Europa, remedio preservativo de muchos males, reparativo de las fuerzas perdidas, y prolongativo de la humana vida."[2] The Iberians did not want to abandon the coca trade but were forced to do so by exterior conditions which posed an exceptional characteristic that persisted until the Victorian Era. The knowledge about proper storage of coca was still not sufficient to transport it overseas and the modes of transportation back then would have taken too long for the plant to arrive on the European continent without losing a significant portion of its potency. If Spain had had the chance to establish a monopoly over the coca trade back then, the history of coca and cocaine certainly would have needed to be rewritten.

1 Acosta, *The Naturall and Morall Historie of the East and West Indies*, 185, 272; Julian, *La Perla de la America*, 39.

2 Julian, *La Perla de la America*, 24, 25; transl.: "Coca could be a highly advantageous branch of commerce for Spain, health of Europe, preservative remedy against many illnesses, restorative of lost forces, and a prolongation of human life."

As with any commodity, people and governments had to be convinced that a new trade article was of value both for the public and the revenue. Resources had to be invested for new commodities, such as personnel and means of transportation while legal regulations concerning taxes or duties had to be negotiated with the other party. Whereas the opium trade could look back on decades of successful business – Opium Wars aside – that flushed plenty of money into the pockets of the British government during the Victorian Era by its revenue, coca started off as a novelty whose marvellous properties were only known to a few. European travellers who ventured to explore South America in the early nineteenth century were the first to report about the benefits of the coca plant and thus introduced British society to a promising new drug. In contrast to Turkish opium, though, which was cultivated in proximity to Britain, coca faced the obstacle of being a commodity which had to be transported across the Atlantic Ocean without losing its power or including massive expenditures on shipping. It was therefore up to the travellers, their experiments, and their reports to indicate the necessity for this trade.

2. Britain's Increasing Interest in Coca

Engaging Europe's attention for such a marvellous plant as the coca shrub was a community effort since it was not specifically a German or Italian who contributed to an increase of awareness but rather several European explorers who all did their fair share to lay the foundation for the coca trade that commenced in the last decades of the nineteenth century. Only the British removed themselves from the equation which contributed to Britain engaging in the coca trade comparatively late and little. I suggest several political, economic, and cultural reasons for that on the following pages.

As mentioned in the previous chapter, Peru and neighbouring countries were part of the Spanish colonial empire until the early nineteenth century. Spain had long been competing with Britain for hegemony but was severely hit by revolutionary uprisings in its colonies in the aftermath of the French revolution. It is possible that Britain refrained from investing money in expeditionary forces to South America during such uncertain times in order not to interfere with the Spanish monopoly and get caught in their wars with the rebels, at least until Peru and other countries gained independence in 1824. Afterwards, sending explorers to investigate a possible expansion of the British imperial realm would also have made little sense since the native population made it clear how they dealt with imperialists. If Spain lost its colonies, there was no point for the British to try and conquer them herself. Apart from that Britain was busy with the opium trade and opium wars in Asia between the 1830s and the early 1860s which caused unexpected expenditures. This could mean that the government – and private organisations anyway – subsequently lacked funding for expeditionary forces to South America as well as motivation to commence trade with yet another narcotic whose medicinal benefits still had to be rediscovered in Europe.

It is safe to say then that the British could rely on first-hand experience in the opium trade whereas in the coca trade, they could not. In the case of opium as the most popular British narcotic, British and Indian physicians, traders, and politicians had the opportunity to witness its production and consumption with their own eyes and draw conclusions they presented in Parliament to channel political action.[3] This contributed to a much more informed assessment of the drug, albeit a biased one. For coca, this was not the case. First reports of the plant and its effects were translations of reports by other European explorers from Germany, Italy, Austria, and France. The descriptions of coca and its consumption also did not appear in widely read and accessible media but rather in specific botanical journals or in several hundred pages long monographs where they could easily be overlooked. In addition, doom-mongering reports such as that of Poeppig did not necessarily increase curiosity in the plant and since only a few European botanists could witness its marvellous properties in situ, their credibility could be doubted. Consequently, Britain had to rely on translated reports for several decades until a sufficient amount made it to the country in 1870 and facilitated experiments with the leaves.

It is not surprising that lacking first-hand encounters with coca and cocaine gave other European countries a head-start in science and trade. In France, a chemist would become a world-renown producer of coca wine after the 1870s and in Germany, several chemists would contribute to make Darmstadt, a city in central Germany, the centre for research in cocaine in the late nineteenth century.[4] Knowing about coca and cocaine's value, they were quick in establishing trade routes with Peru to ensure a consistent supply of the drug and in erecting factories to further process the drugs for consumer

3 Compare HL Deb 12th May 1840, HL Deb 19th March 1858, HL Deb 19th February 1861, HL Deb 3rd August 1894.

4 Gootenberg, *Andean Cocaine*, 57, 58.

markets. Consequently, Britain was already lagging behind economically and in medicinal knowledge before the actual coca trade really started.

3. Establishing a British Coca Trade

Because British cultivation efforts to grow the valuable Peruvian leaf turned out unsuccessful at first, Britain had to look for suitable trading routes with Peru. From 1879 and 1884 the *Guerra del Pacífico* between Peru, Chile, Bolivia impacted trade, but afterwards several dozen steamers and vessels annually plied between Britain and Peru to primarily trade wool, metals, and liquors.[5] Although the Panama Railway connecting the Pacific and Atlantic Ocean via Panama had been completed in 1855, Britain preferred the route around Cape Hoorn (Chile) which was about a five-week journey by ship and less complicated. In the year 1887, 61 British steamers arrived at the Peruvian port of Mollendo via this route and also took the same one home.[6] When records of imported goods to Panama, which was then part of Colombia, became available after 1895, British consuls highlighted that 353 t and 800 t of coca had been transported via the Panama Railway in 1895 and 1896, respectively, but their destinations were unknown.[7]

British consuls in Peru reported about the first coca leaves leaving Peru in 1886 but according to Bills of Entry, exports started earlier than that to supply Britain and other European countries with coca for the manufacturing of coca and cocaine products.[8] Before Niemann's discovery of cocaine in 1859/60 and even in successive years, Bills of Entry often mistook coca for cocoa and vice versa, but the origin of the product and its destination helped to identify the

---

5 House of Commons, *Diplomatic and Consular Reports on Trade and Finance. Peru. Report for the Year 1886 on the Trade of Mollendo* (London: Harrison and Sons, 1887), 1; House of Commons, *Diplomatic and Consular Reports on Trade and Finance. South America. Report for the Year 1887 on the Trade of Mollendo (Peru)* (London: Harrison and Sons, 1888), 2, 3.

6 House of Commons, *Report for the Year 1887 on the Trade of Mollendo (Peru)*, 2.

7 House of Commons, *Diplomatic and Consular Reports on Trade and Finance. Colombia. Report for the Year 1896 on the Trade of Panama* (London: Harrison and Sons, 1897), 32.

8 It is likely that they only reported about Peruvian exports after the war which would explain missing evidence about earlier coca exports. The *Compagnie Maritime au Pacifique*, for example, had established a steamer line between France and Mollendo once a month in 1886, so the route probably had existed before, see House of Commons, *Report for the Year 1887 on the Trade of Mollendo (Peru)*, 2.

correct one.[9] The first amount of coca leaves registered for importation into Britain arrived in Liverpool in 1877 and was an order filled for an unknown recipient. It was just the beginning of the coca trade that would remain on a low, if not insignificant level, until Koller's research on the value of cocaine in ophthalmology presented in 1884 accelerated not only imports but also coca shipments in transit that passed through the port of Liverpool to be delivered to other destinations such as Hamburg, Germany.

There were ten trading posts in Peru of which six were located on the coast (Pacasmayo, Huanchaco, Salaverry, Callao, Pisco, and Mollendo) and four further inlands (Iquitos, Piura, Cerro de Pasco, and Arequipa). The major ports from where coca leaves were exported were Salaverry in the North, Callao, close to Lima, and Mollendo in the South. British ships usually called at the same ports to load and deliver coca, although not exclusively in Peru. The main ports for the British to load coca were Valparaíso in Chile, as well as Salaverry and Mollendo. Other ports such as Callao in Peru, Arica in Chile, and Colón in Panama were also listed but only received smaller amounts for shipment. Ports outside of Peru meant that coca shipments were probably transported there with smaller ships or boats via the Pacific Ocean since the route overland would have taken significantly longer. In addition, it would have impaired the quality of the product since coca lost its potency the longer it was stored. Ships also made several stops on their journey for different commodities, so the last stop to load coca in Valparaíso made sense before they made their journey back to Europe around Cape Hoorn.

The stop in Colón, however, seemed to have been an exception due to its location on the Atlantic Coast. The alternative route via the Panama Railway meant that British ships needed to run between Peruvian ports and Panama City on the Pacific Coast. Coca would then be transported by rail from coast to coast and shipped from the port of Colón to Britain. This route could have taken the British a little over two weeks and thus minimised the shipping time by half, but it was also more complicated since it included different modes of transportation, three additional countries (Panama under Colombian rule, and the US as the constructors of the railway), and therefore higher costs. Until 1900, the route to transport Peruvian coca via Panama to Britain was only cho-

9 Liverpool Customs Bill of Entry, 25th August 1855.

sen in four instances: 12th January 1869, 11th June 1877, 16th September 1885, and 16th July 1887.[10]

The main port of entry for coca leaves in Britain was Liverpool. Until about 1886, the majority of coca that arrived at the port was destined for export to other cities such as Hamburg, Germany which remained the number one export destination until the end of the nineteenth century. In the history of the port, shipments to foreign ports other than Hamburg remained unique incidents, such as the shipment of 105 of serons of coca leaves in transit at Liverpool to New York in 1884.[11] It is likely that coca was transported directly from South to North America afterwards since it was the shorter and more affordable option. In general, there was no regularity in the arrivals of ships from South America having loaded coca. Between 1877 and 1898, 29 different ships with coca and other commodities arrived at Liverpool and only six of them delivered coca to this port more than once during that period. This is interesting because one would think that a continuous supply of raw material was needed to ensure manufacturing of coca products in Britain. The reason can be varying quantities in coca leaves that supplied manufacturers for different lengths of time.

Due to different measurements in the Bills of Entry, it is challenging to determine the exact amounts of coca that entered Britain or that were in transit to other countries. The quantity of coca leaves could be recorded in bales, packages, cases, bags, sacks, or serons ranging in quantity between 1 and 113 during the 1880s and 1890s and even within a singular unit, it was not clear how heavy a bale was, for example.[12] According to an article in the *Planter's Gazette*, coca leaves were primarily packed in bags or small bales, or "more rarely in larger packages weighing 50 or even as much as 60 lbs."[13] In the same month, the Rev-

---

10 Liverpool Customs Bill of Entry, 12th January 1869, 11th June 1877, 16th September 1885, and 16th July 1887.

11 Liverpool Customs Bill of Entry, 5th February 1884. According to Collins Dictionary, a seron (abbreviated srn or srns) is "a bale or parcel wrapped in animal hide, usually containing exotic substances."

12 Liverpool Customs Bill of Entry 23rd November 1877; Liverpool Customs Bill of Entry 24th March 1879, Liverpool Customs Bill of Entry 27th June 1883; Liverpool Customs Bill of Entry 5th October 1883; Liverpool Customs Bill of Entry 25th March 1889; Liverpool Customs Bill of Entry 20th May 1889. In Peru in the 1850s and 1860s, coca leaves were packed in *cestos* à 20 lbs or *tambores* à 50 lbs according to Markham, *Travels in Peru and India*, 235.

13 "Coca," *The Planter's Gazette*, 2nd March 1885, 107.

enue Department of Madras stated that the bags or bales could vary "from 24 to 150 lb."[14] To put that into relation, one can look at imports of another leaf used for indulgence: Unmanufactured tobacco imports into Great Britain in 1900 amounted to roughly 98 million pounds.[15] This certainly makes coca imports appear insignificant but it is safe to say that during that time regular coca trade between South America and Britain existed and that the product was imported into Britain for commercial purposes. The approximate amounts and recipients suggest that this explanation is more likely than those shipments being made on individual orders by wealthy citizens for private consumption.

On most occasions, coca leaves were transported across the ocean upon order by pharmacists or bigger companies. Four companies regularly seemed to have ordered coca from South America, namely Bates, Stokes & Co. from Liverpool, Evans, Sons & Co. and A. Gibbs & Sons from London, and Dawson & Co, also from London. Other companies included Graham Rowe & Co., who were merchants and agents for another company in Lima, Widow Duranty & Son, Japp & Kirby, and Peruvian merchants Duncan, Fox & Co. from Liverpool, Melchers, Runge & Co. from London and Bremen, Braillard Fils & Co. from Paris, as well as J. O. Donnison, T. Davison, T. Williams & Co., Bieber & Co., H. Becker, H. Bright, Rosing Brs. & Co. and J. F. Garagorn.[16] Many of these names usually do not ring a bell – even for anyone knowledgeable about coca products – since they were merely traders or wholesalers in raw materials and not manufacturers. Almost all of them merged with other traders in the twentieth century and often changed their name in the process which makes it difficult to trace their activity back to the Victorian Era.[17]

Among coca trade between South America and Liverpool, a few peculiarities in the Bills of Entry stand out. Until the turn of the century, there was no notion that the purified product, cocaine, had been traded with and there were

---

14 Government of Madras, Revenue Department, 27th March 1885, No. 385; see also: G Bidie, *Coca, its Source, Culture, Uses, &c., (with a Plate)* (Madras: Higginbotham & Co., 1885), 5.

15 The Monopolies Commission, House of Commons, *Report on the Supply of Cigarettes and Tobacco and of Cigarette and Tobacco Machinery* (London: Her Majesty's Stationary Office, 1961), 226.

16 Compare Liverpool Customs Bill of Entry 1855–1899 and London Customs Bill of Entry 1880–1900.

17 The London Archives Collection Catalogue provides information on some of the companies mentioned above and at times also explains their administrative history, https://search.lma.gov.uk/intro.

merely four instances that indicated trade with coca products. In 1894, one case of coca wine arrived in Liverpool but it was marked for export to Trinidad.[18] A year later, three packages and five cases of coca wine were registered for arrival in Liverpool but marked for export to Cape Coast Castle, Ghana in July and November.[19] In 1898, ten cases of coca wine even made it to Belize.[20] The type of product is not too unusual since coca wine enjoyed widespread popularity during the late Victorian Era but that it spread all the way to the Caribbean, Central America, and to Africa is remarkable indeed. Belize, Trinidad, and Ghana were crown colonies at that time and having coca wine transported across such distance indicated a wealthy recipient who was not only willing to pay for it but obviously saw an urgent need to do so. It is possible that the colonies' governors, Sir William Edward Maxwell in Ghana and Sir Frederick Napier Broome in Trinidad were familiar with coca products in Britain and desired to indulge in them when they assumed their roles far away from home.

The assumption of a wealthy recipient is especially true for the unaltered raw coca which was exported to Alexandretta, Turkey and Winnebah, Ghana in 1898.[21] This raises questions about how and why it was consumed there since there is no evidence that there existed factories in either one of these locations which could have manufactured coca products. However, the quantities of 72 and 42 pounds, respectively, would have been sufficient for that purpose. It is not likely that a well-to-do British recipient who could afford shipping of this sort to an overseas destination consumed coca in its original form, i.e., chewing. The only reasonable alternative would have been coca tea. Given its destination, it certainly did not serve the purpose to sustain hunger, labour, or to alleviate altitude sickness, but rather to help with digestive ailments or to act as a reviving tonic.

Besides of a few records of coca products arriving at or transiting through Liverpool, there are no records of any other manufactured coca products, including cocaine, arriving at the port. A British consul in Peru stated that the demand of coca leaves had "sprung up for the manufacture of cocaine," but only 705 quintals (roughly 32,4 t) left the country in 1886 and they were not regis-

18 Liverpool Customs Bill of Entry, 2nd January 1894.

19 Liverpool Customs Bill of Entry, 12th July 1895; Liverpool Customs Bill of Entry, 8th November 1895.

20 Liverpool Customs Bill of Entry, 26th May 1898.

21 Liverpool Customs Bill of Entry, 21st June 1898 and 12th October 1898.

tered for arrival at a British port.[22] The argument that the quantities arriving throughout the year could have been too small to be registered exists but since the Bills of Entry registered even the smallest items on board this contradicts the theory. It is more likely that coca products as well as cocaine were listed under drugs and/or medicine but for obvious reasons, this complicates a better estimate of how much was imported into the country since drugs compromised plenty of other products.

The challenge of varying nomenclature also applied to the port of London where coca leaves arrived as well, but to a much smaller extent and almost exclusively from Hamburg, Germany. Throughout the years between 1880 and 1900, there were just a handful of instances where coca was specifically listed as such.[23] A few more entries list cocoa leaves or cocca leaves which most likely must have been a misspelling of coca leaves. Apart from those minor misspellings, it is questionable what else was coca but not declared as such. Ships arriving from Hamburg carried commodities that were declared as leaves, herbs, drugs, or medicinal spirits that could indicate the raw product or coca products but would also apply to other products, for example camomile and (pepper)mint as leaves and herbs. Nevertheless, some drugs were measured in bales which make those entries stand out. Camomile and peppermint would not have been called drugs, and tobacco, which was well-known, was counted in bales and explicitly labelled as such. Consequently, it is not too far-fetched that the relatively new commodity coca was labelled as a drug and measured in bales since it was comparable to herbs or other leaves and due to the origin of these deliveries in Hamburg. The frequency with which they arrived in London also support this assumption.

This is furthermore confirmed by the increasing entries for imports of bales of drugs for specific years. Before Koller published his research in Heidelberg in 1884 and even one year later, not more than five ships carrying this particular commodity arrived in London from Hamburg annually. But after 1886, deliveries rapidly increased to 26 ships arriving in 1890 that carried bales of drugs. This development is reminiscent of explicitly labelled coca deliveries to the port of Liverpool from Peru which only increased after 1886. The similarities between those two ports in coca and drug deliveries and timing do not

22 House of Commons, *Report for the Year 1887 on the Trade of Mollendo (Peru)*, 2; there are no cocaine listings for the ports of Liverpool or Bristol in that year.

23 London Customs Bill of Entry, 29th July 1885, 218th December 1885, 13th October 1885, 28th November 1900, and 20th December 1900; they were all labelled as cocoa leaves.

seem coincidental. Since after 1890 coca is spelt correctly, it would not be surprising if the customs officers at the port in London needed time to get used to a new commodity that sounded so similar to cocoa and coconuts. Adding to this is the circumstance that Liverpool, rather than London, was the main port of entry for coca and it arrived there in considerable amounts on a somewhat regular basis. A maximum of 97 bales, with an average of about 30 bales, were imported at least once and up to five times a month.[24] Unfortunately, almost all drug shipments counted in bales were marked as orders which makes it difficult to trace them to corresponding recipients.

What is remarkable about coca shipments to the port of London is that they did not come from South America like the ones arriving at Liverpool. Hardly any ships commuted between South America and London, especially not from its West Coast. The few who did commute carried wool, metals, or nitrate sodium. Coca leaves were primarily delivered to London from Hamburg and occasionally from other places such as Madras, Havre, or Trieste.[25] It is likely that more manufactured coca products, rather than raw coca, made it to the port of London which would be included in drugs in general, medicinal spirits, or merchandize. This makes sense insofar as Mariani was the biggest manufacturer of coca products in France and Merck of Darmstadt the biggest manufacturer of cocaine and cocaine products in Europe who could easily transport their products to the Atlantic ports in Havre or Hamburg, respectively, for shipment overseas.

However, there were also statistics that neglected the coca trade altogether. Mulhall wrote in his *Dictionary of Statistics* in 1899, that the "only agricultural exports" from Peru were sugar, wool, and cotton which "show[ed] how backward [...] the condition of the country [was]."[26] For Bolivia, he at least mentioned the coca as a valuable agricultural export product and added that the plant "enabl[ed] travellers to suffer hunger and hardships in so desolate a region."[27] In the first instance, he was outright wrong whereas in the second, he illustrated his ignorance of the value of coca. This is remarkable since by 1899, cocaine had been known for almost four decades and both coca and cocaine products were

---

24 Compare Liverpool Customs Bills of Entry 1877–1899.

25 See, for example, Liverpool Customs Bills of Entry 218th December 1889, 14th November 1895, 3rd May 1900, and 28th November 1900.

26 Michael G Mulhall, *The Dictionary of Statistics* (London: George Routledge and Sons, Ltd., 1899), 48.

27 Ibid.

widely distributed across Britain and Europe. It is surprising that it slipped Mulhall's knowledge that coca's effects were not limited to sustain hunger and hardship and that there existed trade in coca between Peru and Britain. This is especially surprising given that he was a fellow of the Royal Statistical Society and honorary corresponding member of the Royal Scottish Geographical Society who was certainly up to date by reading the news in local papers.[28] Considering the examinations of both the port of London and port of Liverpool, the only way to explain his claim is to assume that his knowledge was limited to trade between the port of London and the world. In this case, his report on British statistics regarding coca would have been at least incomplete.

It is noteworthy that Colombia, which is now the biggest producer of cocaine in the twenty-first century, had hardly any share of the success of coca in the nineteenth century. The British consul in Colombia reported as late as 1888 that the plant was "little grown" and that "[t]he recent demand for coca for the extraction of cocaine [did] not seem to have stimulated its cultivation in any part of the country."[29] There are also no indications that Colombian coca had been traded with between South American countries or that it had left the continent to be shipped overseas. Although assuming a neglectable role in the coca trade back then, the tables rapidly turned after the turn of the century.

4. The German-Peruvian Axis

The transatlantic coca trade, whether between Britain and Peru, or Germany and Peru, was inseparably linked to the production of cocaine. At the end of the nineteenth century, the pharmaceutical industry in Germany was striving and it was thanks to German chemists that it became the centre for cocaine research and the development of new medicine. In winter 1859/60, Albert Niemann first extracted cocaine from coca leaves and in 1884, Carl Koller discovered cocaine's anaesthetic properties which ultimately acted as a juggernaut for the coca trade.[30] The decades in between were not as spectacular for Britain, but it was the golden age of coca products for France and Germany, as explained in Chapter III.

28 Ibid., Title Page.

29 House of Commons, *Diplomatic and Consular Reports on Trade and Finance. Colombia. Report on the Agricultural Condition of Colombia* (London: Harrison and Sons, 1888), 10.

30 Koller, "On the Use of Cocaine for producing Anaesthesia on the Eye."

The shipments in transit via Liverpool to Germany occurred on a somewhat regular basis ranging between one and three times a year between 1885 to 1887 and more regularly, about bi-monthly, between 1894 and 1898.[31] Coca shipments could have also gone directly to the port of Hamburg but it is probable that the ships contained other commodities such as wool that had to be delivered to Britain first before they could continue their journey to Germany. Interestingly, there are no records for coca shipments from Liverpool to Hamburg during the years in between. This indicates that coca was directly transported from Peru to Germany and according to consular reports, the majority of coca from Peru was exported to Hamburg, Germany and amounted to a total of about 300 t in 1898.[32] In contrast to that, only about 9 t were exported to Liverpool. In successive years, the bulk of both coca and cocaine was still exported directly to Germany up to an incredible 922 t in 1903 which was unmatched by exports to any other European or American country.[33]

What comes as a surprise, though, is that after 1902, the destination of coca exports shifted from Europe to the United States. More coca was shipped to North America than to any European country, as was previously the case. Whereas the US solely imported coca leaves in the beginning, Germany continued to import both coca leaves and Peruvian manufactured cocaine, and Britain preferred to import primarily crude cocaine – at least from the port of Salaverry which played a smaller role in the coca trade than Mollendo.[34] The British consul mentioned that there were "21 small factories which manufacture this valuable product [i.e., cocaine, KE]" which could explain why Britain decided to mainly trade with the finished product.[35] Production led to an increase in the price but Britain could eliminate the risk that the leaves lose their potency during shipping and also minimise their effort to produce cocaine at

---

31 Coca shipments to Hamburg passed the port of Liverpool in August 1885, September 1885, February 1886, February 1887, December 1894, March 1895, June 1895, November 1896, March 1897, August 1897, May 1898, July 1898, and September 1898. Compare Liverpool Customs Bill of Entry for those dates.

32 House of Commons, *Diplomatic and Consular Reports. Peru. Report for the Year 1898 on the Trade and Finances of Peru* (London: Harrison and Sons, 1899), 19, 30.

33 House of Commons, *Diplomatic and Consular Reports. Peru. Report for the Year 1902 on the Trade of Peru* (London: Harrison and Sons, 1903), 11, 21; House of Commons, *Diplomatic and Consular Reports. Peru. Report for the Year 1905 on the Trade and General Condition of Peru* (London: Harrison and Sons, 1906), 19.

34 House of Commons, *Report for the Year 1902 on the Trade of Peru*, 28.

35 Ibid., 7.

home. For the US, however, the distance was not as far which could explain their decision to import the raw product for further processing.

The number of German steamers did not increase noteworthy after 1889, but it is likely that the commodities transported back to Germany changed. British consuls in Peru noted that "German steamers did the principal part of the direct shipping from Europe" although only 32 steamers arrived from Germany in contrast to 94 from Britain.[36] Similar to Britain, Germany brought building materials and manufactured goods to Peru in exchange for wool but due to an aspiring pharmaceutical sector, coca became another valuable commodity in their trade. Germany soon realised that it was more profitable to have raw cocaine produced in situ, i.e., Peru, which explained the decreasing amount of coca leaves and the increasing amount of cocaine in the following years.[37]

Nevertheless, coca and cocaine exports were greatly dependent on good harvests and prices were fluctuating. Similar to opium whose price increased 80% in 1886 and again in 1889 due to bad harvests in Asia Minor, coca and cocaine prices increased daily due to bad harvests in Peru and Bolivia in 1890.[38] British consuls in Germany claimed that in this particular year, no coca and cocaine arrived in Germany which further contributed to rising prices.[39] It did not seem, though, as if they lacked continuous supply since in 1892, they reported that there were "abundant supplies of raw material [i.e., coca, KE]" and that the demand for cocaine was "active and business satisfactory."[40] Still, the steady and high demand for cocaine could not disguise the fact that it was

36 House of Commons, *Diplomatic and Consular Reports on Trade and Finance. Peru. Report for the Year 1888 on the Trade of Mollendo* (London: Harrison and Sons, 1889), 2.

37 House of Commons, *Diplomatic and Consular Reports on Trade and Finance. Germany. Report for the Year 1895 on the Trade of Mannheim* (London: Harrison and Sons, 1896), 11.

38 House of Commons, *Diplomatic and Consular Reports on Trade and Finance. Germany. Report for the Year 1886 on the Trade and Agriculture of Wurtemberg* (London: Harrison & Sons, 1887), 6; House of Commons, *Diplomatic and Consular Reports on Trade and Finance. Germany. Report for the Year 1889 on the Trade of the Consular District of Frankfort-on-Maine* (London: Harrison & Sons, 1890), 11.

39 House of Commons, *Diplomatic and Consular Reports on Trade and Finance. Germany. Report for the Year 1890 on the Trade of the District of the Consulate-General at Frankfort* (London: Harrison & Sons, 1891), 14.

40 House of Commons, *Diplomatic and Consular Reports on Trade and Finance. Germany. Report for the Year 1892 on the Trade, &c., of the Grand Duchy of Baden* (London: Harrison & Sons, 1893), 10.

in fact a little profitable business because transport and manufacturing costs were still too high.[41]

As a result, coca products were much more popular and widely available in German-speaking countries and in neighbouring France. Vin Mariani, probably the best-known coca medicine in the nineteenth century, was first advertised in Austrian newspapers in 1872 and experienced a boost in sales with Freud's publication on coca.[42] Reports and advertisement for coca products were published in German-speaking newspapers and magazines from the late 1860s until the beginning of the twentieth century when the International Opium Convention convened in 1912. Shortly before the convention, prices for opium, morphine, and cocaine decreased greatly but this could not prevent the implementation of restrictions to their sales.[43]

In contrast to Britain, Germany started off in the coca business from a more advantageous position. They had explorers who reported about the coca plant from South America as early as the 1810s and, except for Poeppig, were excited about the discovery of such a promising drug. In Germany, coca met with an interested and curious research community that was eager to examine the plant for its medicinal value and that had the means to finance further analysis. Once convinced of its marvellous properties, coca products were manufactured in Germany or imported from France, widely advertised, and had prominent supporters. The success story even amplified when cocaine products concurred with coca products and pharmaceutical companies such as Merck of Darmstadt established a monopoly of cocaine production in Europe, as I explain in a later chapter.

5. The French-Peruvian Axis

Inspired by reports about the marvellous properties of the coca plant and the latest research on cocaine in Germany, a young Corsican pharmacist living in Paris started experimenting with the leaf to develop a medicine that was both

41 House of Commons, *Report for the Year 1892 on the Trade, &c., of the Grand Duchy of Baden*, 10; House of Commons, *Report for the Year 1895 on the Trade of Mannheim*, 8.

42 Allgemeine Wiener medizinische Zeitung 17. (1872), 152, 227; Freud, "Ueber Coca."

43 House of Commons, *Diplomatic and Consular Reports on Trade and Finance. Germany. Report for the Year 1907 on the Trade of the Consular District of Berlin*, (London: Harrison and Sons, 1908), 77.

palatable and conducive to one's health: His name was Angelo Mariani. Fascinated by the research of Mantegazza, Mariani conducted extensive experiments on the effects of coca in hot-houses in Paris.[44] He also established laboratories in Neuilly-sur-Seine, Paris and regularly invited other physicians to visit him to witness the effects of this marvellous plant themselves.[45]

Mariani cultivated a few coca plants there, but he must have gotten a bigger amount of coca leaves for the manufacturing of his products from Peru and Bolivia since he knew about them being of the best quality and containing the highest percentage of alkaloids. The earliest records that coca leaves were transported from the port of Mollendo in Peru to the ports of Havre and Paris in France are from British consuls. In 1898, they reported that a total of about 18 t of coca leaves were shipped which increased to roughly 39 t in 1901.[46] After that year, though, there are no exports to France registered – neither of coca, nor of cocaine. Similarly, it remains unknown how much coca arrived in France before 1898. Diplomatic and consular reports of France in the 1890s only listed drug imports in general that amounted to over 3000 t total.[47] It is likely that the amount of coca was too insignificant to make it on the list of principal articles on its own, or that it was considered insignificant altogether. Unfortunately, it is also difficult to determine how much of the 3000 t they accounted for.[48] Mariani himself stated that the coca leaves he used for his products came "from three different sources and are of incomparable quality," making it likely that he used Peruvian, Bolivian, and lab-grown coca leaves to this end.[49]

However, just as medicine and science rapidly progressed in other European countries after the Industrial Revolution, France grew increasingly cautious of narcotics such as coca. As a result, Vin Mariani was removed from the

44 Mariani, *Coca*, 29, 32–35.

45 Ibid., 4.

46 House of Commons, *Diplomatic and Consular Reports. Peru. Report for the Year 1898 on the Trade and Finances of Peru*, (London: Harrison and Sons, 1899), 19, 30; House of Commons, *Diplomatic and Consular Reports. Peru. Report for the Year 1901 on the Trade and General Condition of Peru* (London: Harrison and Sons, 1902), 26.

47 House of Commons, *Diplomatic and Consular Reports on Trade and Finance. France. Report for the Year 1890 on the Trade of the District of the Consulate General of Havre* (London: Harrison & Sons, 1891), 14.

48 The smallest quantity on the list of imports were rags with 44 t, and in 1898 the quantity was 18 t, so the quantity of coca in previous years must have been below this number.

49 Mariani, *Coca*, 52.

French Pharmaceutical Index in 1910. This was not coincidental with the International Opium Commission that convened in Shanghai in 1909 where various countries pushed for stricter regulations concerning narcotics. Once the biggest customer of French coca products, the United States had become their biggest opponent due to public health concerns and the aspiring temperance movement which caused a big hit to the career of coca, not only in France but in other countries as well.[50] Coca imports into Europe and demands for coca wine decreased rapidly whereas in the US, a guy called John Pemberton introduced his non-alcoholic coca beverage into the market that would become a global success.[51] Slowly but surely, the arrival of Coca-Cola reversed the transatlantic trade of coca products from the pre-existing direction from Europe to North America.

6. Excursus: The British-South Asian Axis

As established in the first chapter, cultivation efforts to grow coca in the British Empire turned out less successful, but Ceylon, nowadays Sri Lanka, seemed to yield the most promising results. Statistics for the export of coca leaves from Ceylon were only available after 1906 but they help to contrast the number of exports of those with South American countries during the same time. Between 1906 and 1909 almost 13 t to 17.4 t of coca leaves were exported from Ceylon, about half of that to Britain and the rest to other European destinations.[52] Whereas this seems quite a lot, it compares unfavourably to the amount of coca leaves exported from Peru, from where 1000 t annually were destined for the German market alone. Even the Dutch who cultivated coca on Java, a former British colony that they still kept themselves well-informed on, exported between 57 t and 465 t during the years 1904–1908.[53] In 1909, less than one percent

50 Gootenberg, *Andean Cocaine*, 191, 192, 207, 208.

51 John Stith Pemberton was the inventor of Coca-Cola in which coca leaves were one of the main ingredients. It might have contained cocaine as well but at the latest in 1908 during a trial between the company and the US government, no amount could be detected in chemical analyses.

52 W H Jackson (Principal Collector) 28th December 1909 in a letter from H Bertram Cox to the Under Secretary of State 10th May 1910.

53 Wyndham R Dunstan, "Memorandum on the Production, Distribution, Sale and Physiological Effects of Cocaine," 16th November 1909, in H Bertram Cox to E Grey, letter, 1st June 1910, TNA.

of these exports were imported into Britain with the majority being shipped to the Netherlands and Germany.[54]

However, the Director of the Imperial Institute pointed out that the coca leaves grown in Java had nothing in common in potency with the Peruvian leaf: "The coca leaves exported from Java contain little or no cocaine, but they are rich in other alkaloids from which cocaine can be made by a comparatively simple process. All the Java coca leaves are at present said to be worked up in Holland for the manufacture of cocaine." [55] Although an analysis by the Royal Botanical Gardens at Kew revealed a cocaine content of up to 0.60% in the Ceylon leaves, it is likely that due to the non-existence of manufacturing companies on the island had to be transported overseas for further processing. This exacerbated smooth trade and sales of coca and products thereof on the British market which is one of the reasons why Britain eventually decided to primarily import the South American leaf and (crude) cocaine after the turn of the century.

The trade between Britain and Ceylon was not limited to exports from the latter to the former but also included the import of cocaine into British India and the Straits Settlements. Like statistics on coca trade with Indian and East Indian territories, statistics on cocaine were only available at the beginning of the twentieth century. Between 1904 and 1908, Britain imported between 35 and 112kg of cocaine annually into British India, with additional neglectable amounts being imported from Belgium and Germany.[56] Letters between Governor John Anderson to the Under Secretary of State at the Foreign Office in Britain, wired through the Earl of Crewe and H Bertram Cox, also mentioned concerns over imports of cocaine into the Straits Settlements: "[...] [T]he evils resulting from morphine and cocaine injections are immeasurably greater in intensity and extent [than that of opium, KE] [...] [W]e are[,] I regret to say[,] making no real progress towards an effective diminution in the evil."[57] Despite realising that cocaine, just like opium and morphine, was a dangerous narcotic, this statement indicates that Britain had not learnt from the spread of the opium and morphine habit in British India to limit or abstain from cocaine imports into the country altogether.

54 Ibid.

55 Ibid.

56 Memorandum of the Director of the Imperial Institute in a letter from H Bertram Cox to the Under Secretary of State 1st June 1910.

57 John Anderson to the Under Secretary of State, 30th March 1910, letter, TNA.

Instead, the poor handling of the narcotics trade, including the delayed response to the spread of addiction in various territories and insufficient restrictions on behalf of government officials, led to an increase of illicit trafficking even before political regulations came into effect. This was mostly evident in the Straits Settlements. In Singapore and Penang for the first five months of 1910, 9,168 and 3,848 bottles of cocaine were seized, respectively.[58] Whereas a majority seemed to have been of German origin, being marked E Merck of Darmstadt, the primary producer of cocaine at the time, the rest were marked Lin Kee, London. The superintendent suspected that this brand was "fictitious" and highlighted that a lot of smuggling took place through British ports which required action.[59] One reason for this smuggling strategy could have been to avoid taxes or duties on imports, but it is also possible that a rebranding of cocaine and products thereof increased accessibility and acceptance in foreign customers.

Although Britain also exported cocaine to China, they took a different approach to its trade than a few decades prior in the opium trade. Rather than ignoring Chinese edicts and using military force to enforce their interest as in the Opium Wars, Britain decided to adhere to China's regulations concerning the prohibition of cocaine imports into the country for other than medicinal purposes, as the consul of Amoy stated: "I do not anticipate any objections on the part of British merchants to this prohibition – although cocaine has become [...] a favourite commodity among the southern Chinese. Large quantities are brought into this port [...]."[60] In Canton, the situation was seemingly different as the consul there argued that "[...] cocaine is not imported by British firms."[61] Eventually, Müller issued a copy of the King's regulations to the Straits Settlements prohibiting them from 1st December 1910 to import cocaine and instruments for its injection into China, and manufacturing cocaine there.[62] These became known as "The Cocaine Prohibition Regulations."

The evidence concerning British coca and cocaine trade with and in South Asia suggests that Britain did not pursue a different approach depending on whether the trading countries were part of the imperial realm or not. Britain's

58 F M Baddeley to the Colonial Secretary of the Straits Settlement, 1st June 1910, letter, TNA.

59 Baddeley to the Colonial Secretary of the Straits Settlement, 1st June 1910.

60 Amoy consul to W G Max Müller, 30th June 1910, letter, TNA.

61 Canton consul to W G Max Müller, 11th July 1910, letter, TNA.

62 W G Max Müller to the consuls of the Straits Settlements, 11th October 1910, letter, TNA.

history with China in the opium trade certainly guided their approach when they refrained from their imperialistic attitude, that was still evident in the early and mid-nineteenth century, in respecting China's regulations concerning the import of coca and cocaine. This fostered sympathetic trade connections and illustrated Britain's position in the international narcotics trade that became increasingly relevant at the beginning of the twentieth century.

Similarly, coca and cocaine imports into British India from Britain did not by far reach the extent of opium imports a few decades earlier and restrictions were put in place rather quickly. As the members of the Cocaine Committee explained: "[...] in India, importation by post is prohibited, importation by other channels is severely restricted, and possession by private persons is forbidden, except under the authority of a medical prescription."[63] Given that the International Opium Conference in The Hague 1911/12 took place before this report was written and submitted, it can be assumed that the latter was a result of the former.

7. Differing Attitudes

It is obvious that the transatlantic coca trade and the trade with cocaine in Europe were overlapping since the time between the import of significant amounts of coca, the development of coca medicine, and the discovery of cocaine was compromised to only a few decades. The developments in medicine and science in the Victorian Era allowed coca to experience a much more accelerated career than opium but at the same time it had to face opposition given the rather short time for adequate trials. In Germany, this circumstance did not matter too much since it was about to become the centre of chemical and pharmaceutical research in Europe and could not afford to lose time with tedious trials. But in Britain, the situation was different since the country looked back on a long history of narcotic trade with Asia and of narcotic consumption at home that influenced their attitude towards new drugs on the market.

One reason for Britain's cautious attitude towards coca was the lack of first-hand witnesses of the marvellous plant of the Andes: No British explorer or traveller or significant personality could confirm or reject notions that coca

63 Cocaine Committee to the Colonial Secretary, "Opium, Morphia, and Cocaine," 29th August 1912, report, TNA.

indeed sustained hunger and labour which could therefore be valuable to the vast working population back home. Britain had to rely on translations well until the late Victorian Era when coca experiments were facilitated by sufficient imports. It does not come as a surprise then that the initial reaction to coca in Britain was much more muted than in Germany or France, especially when considering the economic challenges of coca procurement.

Even when well-known researchers such as Sir Christison confirmed that coca leaves were of medicinal value and cocaine had been discovered, Britain did not officially pick up on the chance to become a major player in the coca trade. From the outside, it seemed like merely another drug in a row of plenty to choose from.[64] However, botanical reports reveal that Britain in fact knew about coca's potential as a drug, but Germany and France already had a foot in the door with their progress in coca research and the development of coca products. After Kew experienced mostly unsuccessful cultivation efforts across the Empire, Britain decided not to enter a serious competition with their European neighbours in the trade. This is confirmed by the importation of coca into Britain which was rather irregular in terms of shipments, quantities, and trading companies. For decades, the opium trade had already been a lucrative but challenging drug business for Britain that possibly made it unattractive to engage in yet another drug trade.

Given the rising popularity of both coca and cocaine products, there was also no need for that. The pharmaceutical industry in Britain quickly realised their opportunity to draw a profit from these products through clever advertising in newspapers which played into the hands of profit-oriented businessmen. Some products, like *Vin Mariani*, were imported from the continent but at the end of the nineteenth century, pharmacists, chemists, and druggists had developed their own recipes for coca medicine. Among them Hall's Coca Wine and cocaine pastilles from Allen & Hanbury, both located in central London, who regularly advertised their products. British companies chose to focus their effort on importing the final products rather than engaging in overseas trade and manufacturing like Germany and France.

These explanations seem especially true since the discovery of cocaine as the first local anaesthetic in 1884 did not make a significant difference in the trade of coca with South American countries. Although more coca was

64 Other popular drugs included herbs such as camomile and peppermint, but also more concerning ones such as opium, morphine, henbane, belladonna, and strychnine.

imported from Peru after that date, specifically labelled imports of the purified product cocaine were singular incidents. In fact, there was only one instance in the nineteenth-century history of the port of Liverpool when a box of cocaine made it into the country, and during the same time only one case of cocaine made it to the port of London.[65] It is possible, though, that cocaine was imported under the umbrella term 'drugs' or 'merchandize' which complicates concrete statements as to the origin, quantity, and regularity of cocaine imports into Britain. Consequently, a precise quantification of the coca trade between South America and Britain at that time is impossible but it existed, nonetheless.

In any way, the economic stage in the trajectory of coca in Victorian Britain evolved naturally from the botanical stage and laid the groundwork for further medicinal trials that resulted in coca medicine being developed by the pharmaceutical industry. Now that trade with coca and later cocaine was established, the pharmaceutical industry in Britain could focus on marketing those two novel narcotics and making them available for the public. As the next chapter shows, this equally came with its challenges that would eventually result in political action to restrict the sale and consumption not only in the home country but in the colonies as well.

65 Bill of Entry Liverpool, 8th October 1895; Bill of Entry London, 21st February 1900.

Chapter III: Marketing a Marvel

1. Medical Marvels

When we think of 'medical marvels' in the Victorian Era, we think of new drugs on the market that possessed specific effects that had never been seen before and that significantly changed the health of a patient. Often these discoveries occurred when raw products were purified but the purification alone did not always act as a juggernaut for the career of a particular drug. This was especially true for coca whose purified product cocaine did not evoke immediate euphoria but required other circumstances to vault it into the league of narcotic superstars.[1] In fact, the most important among those circumstances was a changed mode of consumption, or rather, changed mode of administration which had a huge impact on the potency of these narcotics.

In the 1870s and 1880s, the medical profession took an increased interest in the medicinal value of coca which later included that of its alkaloid cocaine.[2] Coca was advertised as the best tonic for singers and it proved a much better remedy for gastrointestinal ailments than opium since it neither produced indigestion, nor did it come with any other notable side effects. The exceptionality in a medicinal context, though, came with the discovery of cocaine as the first local anaesthetic. It was much more reliable, safer, and easier to administer than other anaesthetics at the time – such as ether and chloroform – and

1 These circumstances included sociocultural developments, as will be examined in the next chapter.

2 Compare, for example, Alexander Bennett, "The Physiological Action of Coca," *British Medical Journal* (18th April 1874): 510; Robert Christison, "Observations on the Effects of Cuca, or Coca, the Leaves of Erythroxylon Coca," *British Medical Journal*, vol. 1 no. 800 (29th April 1876): 527–531; and Koller, "On the Use of Cocaine for Producing Anaesthesia on the Eye."

led to a revolution in surgery.[3] Additional experiments also confirmed its use as a mood elevator which later contributed to its recreational use.

From a pharmaceutical point of view, coca and cocaine were also exceptional because they could be offered in a variety of forms for a wide range of conditions. In a way, this resembled opium products and their applications, so it was a decisive factor in profit-making. However, in contrast to opium and other drugs on the market, coca and cocaine products were not affordable for the working class and primarily used by the upper classes.[4] They were luxury products that only became a common commodity in the first decades of the twentieth century when political restrictions on the drugs limited accessibility in a different way.

2. Pharmaceutical Networking

When coca entered the pharmaceutical sphere, the role of Kew as the centre of research on coca diminished significantly. Kew as a botanical institution was the facilitator for experimental research on the plant that could lead to the creation of medicine, but it did not have sufficient connections in the pharmaceutical sector that could have justified a continuance of their previously eminent role. Nevertheless, connections outside of the Kew network and particularly in other European countries, for example between chemists and physicians, chemists and wholesalers, or among physicians produced valuable outcomes for coca's career in general.

In contrast to botanists and Kew, who had an employer-employee relationship, other ties were in rarer instances constructed of friendship. A friendship such as between Angelo Mariani and Dr Charles Fauvel in France, for example, had the potential to blur the lines between business and friendship that could as well develop from one another.[5] Dr Charles Fauvel, who was an expert

3 "Hydrochlorate of Cocaine, the new local Anaesthetic," *British Medical Journal* (29th November 1884), 1081; "Cocaine," *Chambers's Journal of Popular Literature, Science and Arts* 3, no. 114 (6th March 1886), 145, 147.

4 As Picard stated in "The working class and the poor:" "A labourer's wage averaged between 20 and 30 shillings a week in London, probably less in the countryside. This would just cover his rent, and a very sparse diet for him and his family;" A bottle of coca wine from Allen & Hanbury's still cost 2 shillings and 6 dimes in 1908 which would have been a worker's daily wage, see *General List of Drugs*, 165.

5 "Dr Charles Fauvel," *British Medical Journal*, Vol. 1 (11th January 1896), 118.

in pharyngology, could test Mariani's coca products on his patients and thus make recommendations concerning their applications. Mariani then used this knowledge to advertise his products and use Fauvel's popularity to promote them. In turn, Fauvel could prescribe Mariani's coca products to his patients which must have been financially profitable for both. In *Coca and its Therapeutic Applications*, Mariani wrote that the "eminent specialist" Fauvel "[...] specifies Mariani's extract of Coca leaves in preference to solutions of Cocaine [...]" and declared Vin Mariani a "Tensor of the vocal cords."[6] Of course, there were no notions of their friendship in those publications to avoid rumours about nepotism and Fauvel's name was only one among many other physicians who testified for Mariani.

A blurring of the lines between chemistry and medicine could also be witnessed in Germany, especially after the discovery of cocaine but before its hypodermic application. Psychiatrist Freud, for example, was friends with ophthalmologist Koller who also had connections to neurologist Mantegazza in Italy. Freud and Koller became friends when they both worked and resided at the General Hospital in Vienna which led to several experiments with cocaine.[7] Unfortunately for Freud, he was out of the country when his friend achieved the breakthrough with cocaine as a local anaesthetic in ophthalmology. Later, his essay "Ueber Coca" left him branded as an addicted psychoanalyst until today.

Manufacturing chemists did not only establish ties with physicians but also with wholesalers or traders in coca who ensured the supply of the drug in Britain. Graham Rowe & Co, for example, were agents in Lima, Peru who were employed by merchants and bankers Frederick Huth, Gruning & Co in the 1870s. Charles Graham Rowe was born in Lima and by the 1880s, the company imported coca through the port of Liverpool. This mutual relationship facilitated coca exports since it combined the expertise of personnel in situ, i.e., that of Peruvian-born agents who knew about the quality of different kinds of coca and the mechanisms of coca trade before it left the country, and the expertise of the merchants who enabled overseas trade and took care of the goods entering British ports.

During the Victorian Era, professions were not yet as sharply distinguished as they are today which caused some ambiguity between druggists,

6 Mariani, *Coca and its Therapeutic Applications*, 46, 55, 56.

7 Angerer, "Carl Koller,inscribed on reverse: Seinem lieben Freund Dr Sigmund Freud. April 1885 Dr Carl Koller," photograph, April 1885, Freud Museum, London, https://www.freud.org.uk/collections/archives/archive-records/IN/1510/.

pharmacists, chemists, and pharmaceutical chemists.[8] They all had knowledge in chemistry and pharmacy but with specific emphasis depending on their jobs. Until 1868, everyone could call themselves one of these professions, even quacks, until the Pharmacy Act ruled that people manufacturing and dispensing medicine had to undergo examinations to be properly licensed to do so. This ensured a certain standard in the business that consumers could rely on, and it contributed to increased safety in public health. Nevertheless, professions in the pharmaceutical sector greatly contributed to the success of coca and cocaine in the last decades of the nineteenth century.

3. Research on Coca

Italian neurologist and anthropologist Paolo Mantegazza, who worked in South America in the 1850s, was among the first and few who reported extensively about coca through self-experimenting which was a driving force for the scientific interest in the plant in Europe. Similar to explorers who witnessed the effects of coca before him, he was surprised that knowledge about it had not reached Europe with the Spaniards but had largely been forgotten for almost three centuries.[9] He therefore regarded it as his duty "che se ne studii l'azione fisiologica, che se ne pesino i vantaggi e pericoli, che se ne limiti con esattezza il confine terapeutico, che si cherchi infine di metter di contro i trovati della tradizione popolare coi risultati della scienza, per vedere fino a dove e in che combaciano."[10]

Mantegazza consumed coca daily for about two years as coca tea and by mastication in varying amounts. His results matched with the effects witnessed in the indigenous population, namely that it was a stimulant that gave strength to its consumers and acted as a remedy against gastrointestinal illnesses regardless of age or race wherefore he considered it safe to use for everyone in moderation.[11] Nevertheless, he also warned about its dangers that

8 S W F Holloway, *Royal Pharmaceutical Society of Great Britain, 1841–1991, A Political and Social History* (London: The Pharmaceutical Press, 1991), 83, 84.

9 Mantegazza, *Quadri della natura umana*, 510, 511.

10 Mantegazza, *Quadri della natura umana*, 522, transl.: "that the physiological action is studied, the advantages and dangers weighed, the therapeutic boundaries limited with precision, that the findings of popular traditions are contrasted with scientific results to finally see where they match."

11 Ibid, 495, 496.

he experienced himself. In a state of fantasmagoria, he noted down his most popular and often cited quote, that he preferred "una vita di 10 anni con coca che una di 100000..... (e qui seguiva una riga di zeri) secoli senza coca."[12] Mantegazza was aware that the chemical composition of coca was still unknown but argued that this was also true for opium and its mode of operation. Being convinced of coca's value as a therapeutic, he encouraged Europeans to raise it on the same level as opium since it was a "vero tesoro del Nuevo Mondo."[13] Unfortunately, as Sigmund Freud later observed, "[s]eine Mittheilung hat viel Aufmerksamkeit erregt, aber wenig Vertrauen gefunden."[14]

It was not until 1859 that enough coca leaves arrived in Europe for further scientific investigation with the Austrian ship *Novara* that had been on a journey around the world for the previous three years. In von Wüllerstorf-Urbair's report that was published in 1862, he explained that he brought 30 pounds of coca leaves back with him, and a little later two German colleagues living in Lima sent him an additional 30 pounds.[15] Given the year of the publication, Wüllerstorf-Urbair was already aware how significant his delivery was to humanity since Albert Niemann had extracted the valuable alkaloid cocaine shortly after his arrival back home.[16] Realising that the coca leaves had lost most of their potency on their overseas journey but that they were of extraordinary importance for medicinal developments in Europe, he was convinced that "[es] dürften sich leicht Mittel finden lassen, um den wirksamen Stoff der Coca in ähnlicher Weise sofort an Ort und Stelle aus den Blättern zu extrahieren."[17]

Rather than being repulsed by Poeppig's report but inspired by von Tschudi, Weddell, and Mantegazza, British physician Sir Robert Christison from the University of Edinburgh was curious as well to experiment with the leaf himself. According to Christison, "a London mercantile gentleman, Mr. Batchelor" brought him coca leaves and a coca plant from Peru in 1864 but it was not until 1870 that he started experimenting with them.[18] It would take

12 Ibid., 493, transl.: "a life of ten years with coca to more than 100.000 ... [...] without it."

13 Ibid., 496.

14 Freud, "Ueber Coca," 294.

15 *Reise der Oesterreichischen Fregatte Novara um die Erde, in den Jahren 1857, 1858, 1859 unter den Befehlen des Commodore B. von Wüllerstorf-Urbair. Beschreibender Theil. Dritter Band* (Wien: Kaiserlich-Königliche Hof- und Staatsdruckerei, 1862), 348.

16 Ibid.

17 Ibid., 352, transl.: "it should be easy to gather the means to extract the active principle of the coca plant in situ in a similar manner."

18 Christison, "Observations on the Effects of Cuca," 528.

another six years until he presented his findings before the Botanical Society of Edinburgh in April 1876 which were then published in the *British Medical Journal* two weeks later. The amount of coca leaves simply were not sufficient to provide reliable results.[19] Christison then received more coca from Sir Charles Wyville Thomas, a fellow professor in Edinburgh who accompanied the *Challenger* expedition from 1872 to 1876, and from Dr Alexander Bennett, son of Professor John Hughes Bennett in Edinburgh, who brought them from Paris to use the leaves for his experiments with animals.[20]

Although he was the first known British professional to undertake a more detail survey on the effects of coca and publish it, Christison's experiments were limited. They were confined to chewing coca during long walks that he and some of his students made in London and during two hikes up Ben Vorlich, a 3,224 ft tall mountain, with his son.[21] He concluded that coca chewing "remove[d] extreme fatigue, and prevente[d] it. Hunger and thirst [we]re suspended; but eventually appetite and digestion [we]re unaffected."[22] Nevertheless, as an experienced and well-trained physician that he was, he reminded the audience that he could neither draw conclusions about the effects of a coca habit nor return a verdict about its usefulness in medicine.[23]

Despite the limitations of Christison's experiments, a few things stand out. First, it is remarkable that the coca leaves he consumed were still potent enough for him to witness any effects. Storing and shipping times must have improved significantly over the previous decades for this to be the case. Also, the availability must have improved and the price dropped (at least to a certain extent) for him to consider acquiring coca leaves. In addition, Christison was aware that he needed to level the playing-field to experience the same effects as Peruvian coca chewers. Britain certainly did not provide him with similar altitudes as the Andes in South America to prove the alleviating effects on altitude sickness – although Ben Vorlich seemed to be tall enough for the average urban Victorian – but he realised that he needed to exhaust himself enough to witness coca's sustaining powers. At that time, Christison was already 78 years old but still went on long walks and hikes to satisfy his wanderlust.

---

19 Ibid., 527.

20 Christison, "Observations on the Effects of Cuca," 527, 529; G H Brown, "Alexander Hughes Bennett," *The Times*, 5th November 1901.

21 Christison, "Observations on the Effects of Cuca," 529, 530.

22 Ibid., 530.

23 Ibid., 530, 531.

4. The Discovery of Cocaine

Being preeminent in his field as the president of the British Medical Profession, Christison was convinced that no one before him had conducted experiments with coca leaves in Britain. This is remarkable since cocaine had been discovered as early as 1859 but did not spark as much curiosity in the British medical world even in 1876, when he gave his speech. Christison only briefly mentioned that a "crystalline principle" had been found but preferred not to conduct a chemical analysis. Ironically, him doing so and conducting further experiments would have meant a breakthrough in the success of the drug in Britain. It would have enabled pharmacists to purify coca themselves and conduct further experiments with the alkaloid as to the effects on the human body.

There is some disagreement whether Niemann was the first to discover cocaine due to Friedrich Gaedcke's research five years earlier in 1854. In contrast to Niemann, Gaedcke was a pharmacist in Rostock and the impact of his research was limited. A merchant called Worlée supplied Gaedcke with two ounces of coca leaves for his experiments from which he wanted to prove that coca contained a crystalline substance which was similar to theïn found in tea.[24] After unsuccessful experiments, he eventually managed to extract a crystalline substance but the amount did not suffice for purification and to arrive at a conclusion. Nevertheless, Gaedcke named the substance *Erythroxylin* and explained that further experiments with a higher amount of coca were required to confirm his findings.[25] Unfortunately for him, Gaedcke suffered the fate of many pharmacists who lacked the popularity and means to expand and publish their studies, wherefore the discovery of cocaine was not attributed to him.

Instead, it was another researcher in Göttingen who carried off the laurels in the winter of 1859/60. It was Albert Niemann, a PhD student in chemistry at the University of Göttingen under supervision of Prof Friedrich Wöhler. Niemann's place of work played a crucial role in the discovery of cocaine: His supervisor supplied him with fresh coca leaves from the expedition of the Novara to conduct experiments in search of alkaloids.[26] Niemann first soaked coca leaves in a mixture of 85% alcohol and sulfuric acid to dissolve particles from

24 Gaedcke, *Ueber das Erythroxylin*, 9, 14.

25 Ibid., 14.

26 Albert Niemann, *Über eine neue organische Base in den Cocablättern* (Göttingen: E A Huth, 1860), 7.

the leaves during a four-day digestion at 40° Celsius.[27] The leaves were then pressed and the process repeated. Afterwards, Niemann added hydrated lime, neutralised the tincture with sulfuric acid, and through distillation separated alcohol from a resinous substance.[28] He repeatedly mixed this substance with water to obtain a solution that he would unite with the first filtration.[29] To test whether this mixture indeed contained alkaloids, he added sodium carbonate which produced precipitation in the test tube. In conjuncture with ether, Niemann shook it and skimmed the resulting layer which was then distilled. As a result, the residue developed into a crystalline mass that only had to be purified to dispose of the colour and voilà: cocaine was extracted.[30] Niemann later published his experiments on cocaine as a dissertation which fostered his popularity and caused him to be attributed with its discovery.

Niemann's method of extracting cocaine from raw coca was challenging, so at the end of the nineteenth century, crude cocaine, a kind of paste from coca leaves, was produced in coca-originating countries and shipped to Europe for further processing. Burroughs and Wellcome's recipe books describe this process in great detail.[31] At first, Ecgonine methyl ester hydrochloride had to be created from a mixture of crude cocaine, methyl alcohol, and sulphuric acid. Afterwards, this was turned into cocaine hydrochloride which, after additional chemical treatment, was turned into cocaine in its crystalline form. The extraction process involved several chemicals that included "'Shell' Motor Spirit," chloroform, and various types of alcohol and took several days.[32] Cocaine prices remained high until the turn of the century as the raw material was still scarce and the manufacturing process complex.

From a modern point of view, it seems as if cocaine itself was the marvel that "flashed like a meteor before the eyes of the medical world" but this was only half the truth. Coca's alkaloid certainly brought with it an increased potency and thus an extended range of applications but it was far away from what

27 Ibid., 27, 28.

28 Ibid., 28.

29 Ibid., 29.

30 Ibid., 30.

31 Chemical Department, *Processes* (Burroughs, Wellcome & Co, 1908). As the author noted for the extraction of cocaine: "The hydrochlorides of the total alkaloids are hydrolysed and the hydrochlorides of ecgonine are pseudotropine from the non-alkaloid matter. They are converted to methyl ester, heated with benzoyl chloride and the cocaine separated from the tropacocaine by the treatment with ammonia."

32 Chemical Department, *Processes*, "Shell" in quotation marks in the original.

happened after 1884. On 17th October, a young ophthalmologist from Vienna called Carl Koller presented the findings of his latest research at the ophthalmologic congress in Heidelberg – it would revolutionise medicine.[33] Koller had experimented with cocaine and realised that it possessed anaesthetic properties which made eye surgeries much safer and easier. But what was an anaesthetic for the eye was also an anaesthetic for other parts of the body and in contrast to the popular chloroform and ether, cocaine became the very first *local* anaesthetic. Koller's discovery was proof that medical marvels did not merely refer to the purified drugs but that they were marvellous because a changed mode of administration made their full potency visible. As the *British Medical Journal* observed: "Had it not been for his [Koller's, KE] energy and enterprise, the peculiar physiological properties of this valuable alkaloid might have remained in oblivion for another twenty years."[34] The field of medicine in the Victorian Era was not in its infancy anymore, yet it still had to rely on trial and error to determine the amounts of narcotics that crossed the line from useful to dangerous and potentially deadly drugs.

This ambivalence in opinions over cocaine was reinforced when hypodermic syringes opened the door for new applications of the drug. Syringes had been in use since the 1850s but they were mostly used in general practices and by the upper classes who were able to afford the treatment as they were still very expensive. The subcutaneous administration of cocaine greatly increased its potency since the drug was no longer absorbed by tissue before it could unfold its full effect. Whereas this mode of administration was much quicker than oral consumption, the fastest and at the same time most dangerous mode was intravenous where cocaine entered the bloodstream instantaneously. Due to a lack of adequate trials, this often led to patients dying from accidental poisoning by their doctors and even they themselves occasionally faced the same fate during self-trials. Trials on animals such as those of Alexander Bennett and Ralph Stockman proved only partially helpful which had the former admit that "of [cocaine's] beneficial action in medical practice [he was] not yet in a position to give an opinion."[35] Knowledge about the effects of different modes

---

33 "Hydrochlorate of Cocaine, the new local Anaesthetic," *British Medical Journal* (29th November 1884), 1081.

34 "Cucaine and its salts," *British Medical Journal* (13th December 1884), 1201–1.

35 Bennett, "The Physiological Action of Coca," 510; Stockman, "Report on the Coca Alkaloids," 1043.

of administration and potentially deadly amounts of cocaine were still obscure and even among professionals, opinions varied.[36]

In an *Inquiry into the Questions of Deaths resulting from the Administration of Anaesthetics* from 1910, for example, physicians and coroners agreed that the application of cocaine was "still in its infancy," wherefore ether and chloroform continued to be the favoured form of anaesthesia.[37] Because or despite of little knowledge about cocaine and its role in accidental deaths, they suggested no "legislative interference" and recommended its administration only by qualified physicians.[38] The coroners remarked that more research still needed to be done in anaesthesia to find the perfect anaesthetic agent but in saying so, they lacked the understanding that there was no drug that fitted all purposes or all people, just as there was no one size fits all regarding its dose. This stood in contrast to the knowledge of pharmacists who were well aware of this circumstance, as I explain later.

Despite of the advancement of medicinal knowledge accidental poisonings from narcotics such as cocaine did not decrease over time because potentially doses were still unknown. Even if cocaine was administered by a professional, for example a dentist, poisoning could not be excluded and sometimes led to lawsuits in which a patient's family sued the doctor, as in Farvish v. Zeifert.[39] In addition, syringes became cheaper and more widely available and patients could freely obtain their desired drug from the pharmacy around the corner. This facilitated self-administration that was rarely monitored by a physician and increased chances of accidental poisoning and even death. Consequently, medical professionals regularly warned that cocaine "may be toxic, sometimes deadly," especially "when given under the skin."[40]

Therefore, the purification of coca in the form of cocaine was not sufficient as a booster for narcotic consumption and cannot claim to be the marvel many have talked about. Instead, it was the hypodermic application that suddenly

---

36 "The estimated minimum lethal dose of cocaine is 1.2g," Amy Sue Biondich and Jeremy David Joslin, "Coca: The History and Medical Significance of an Ancient Andean Tradition," *Emergency Medicine International* (2016), 2.

37 Coroner's Committee, House of Commons, *Report of Inquiry Into the Question of Deaths Resulting from the Administration of Anaesthetics* (London: Eyre and Spottiswoode, 1910), 5, 6.

38 Coroner's Committee, *Report of Inquiry*, 6.

39 "Inquest. Cocaine for Tooth Extraction," *The Times* (23rd January 1908), 5.

40 J B Mattison, "Cocaine Dosage and Cocaine Addiction," *The Lancet* (21st May 1887), 1024, 1026.

changed a potent narcotic into a potentially deadly narcotic. The effects did not occur slowly and somewhat comprehensible anymore but instantaneous and incontrollable. Neither the medical profession nor the pharmacists could keep up with this development in knowing fatal doses for this new mode of administration which increased risks for patients. As marvellous as hypodermic injections of cocaine were for the revolution of surgeries, they also opened pandora's box which led to increased cases of addiction and the creation of a modern menace.

5. Coca(ine) for the Public

Although the contact between societies in history produced a change in cultural practices, coca chewing has continued to be the primary mode of consumption for centuries. Together with drinking coca tea it has remained the most popular method in Peru until this day. However, chewing coca was not becoming for the average Victorian as it was considered an indigenous habit and was frowned upon like gum chewing today. As a tea-loving country, they also had better alternatives to coca tea such as Darjeeling, Ceylon or Assam tea that would produce much better effects due to their high levels of caffeine. Still, the marvellous property of coca to prevent fatigue lured some people to experiment with the leaves to find alternative forms of consumption.

One result of experimentation with coca was coca wine, most prominently produced and advertised by Angelo Mariani as *Vin Mariani*. For his precious and soon-to-become popular wine, he soaked the leaves in high quality Bordeaux wine and presented his product to the public for the first time in 1863. In the beginning, Mariani promoted his coca wine as a remedy against pharyngeal and laryngeal illnesses but he also realised its potential as a remedy against ailments of the digestive system.[41] Soon news circulated about this new medicine that was praised both a remedy for sore throats of professional singers and a refreshing tonic which led to Mariani's first shop being opened in Paris in 1880. Just four years later, his invention made it into the French Pharmaceutical Codex and about the same time, his product was popular across Europe

41 Mariani, *Coca and its Therapeutic Applications*, 44–48. Pharyngeal and laryngeal illnesses affect the pharynx and/or larynx, e.g. problems with the vocal cords, infections, tonsillitis, throat cancer.

and made it across the ocean all the way to the United States. One of *Vin Mariani's* most famous consumers was US President Ulysses S. Grant who was given the medicine to alleviate pains accompanying throat cancer. Hundreds of other consumers, including Pope Leo XIII. who awarded him the Vatican gold medal, all greatly recommended *Vin Mariani* and contributed to the product becoming a global success. Mariani's coca wine was only the beginning of a global success story that later inspired American pharmacist John Pemberton to invent a drink that became known as Coca-Cola.

As the popularity of *Vin Mariani* increased, copycats jumped on the bandwagon to create their own coca wine and engage in competition with the brand leader. There was Armbrecht's coca wine, Hall's coca wine, Jesse William's coca wine, Comaltana Wine, Marza Wine, and Vinacoca who competed for customers and forced Mariani to expand his product range. He added not only another liquid coca preparation – an elixir – but also pâte, thé, and pastilles to his assortment. The original *Vin Mariani* contained about 0,2g of cocaine in a litre, amounting to a cocaine content of approximately 0,02%. Coca leaves in alcohol dissolve the cocaine from the leaves wherefore its content was higher in liquors than in watery solutions. According to Mariani, the *Elixir Mariani* was "more alcoholic" and "three times as highly charged with the aromatic principles of the Coca leaf as the *Vin Mariani*," which would account for a cocaine content of roughly 0,06%.[42] The *Pâtes Mariani*, or lozenges, were "[c]omposed only of clarified gum, sugar and Coca," which made them the weakest coca products in Mariani's product range, together with *Thé Mariani*.[43] Lozenges and tea in general are still consumed in Peru as remedies against altitude sickness or un-wellbeing and are not subject to any restrictions regarding their sale or consumption.

In Germany, the popularity of specific coca products looked somewhat different since coca pills were the more sought-after product. This development was greatly influenced by products manufactured by Dr Sampson and Dr Alvarez who regularly promoted their pills for a variety of ailments in public newspapers after 1870. Dr Sampson was a physician from New York who worked closely with Dr Schulze in Berlin and Braunschweig and most likely came across coca in his homeland where the drug was on the rise. His product range consisted of three kinds of pills of which *Coca-Pillen I* helped with chest pains, *Coca-Pillen II* battled abdominal pain, and *Coca-Pillen III* strengthened

42 Mariani, *Coca and its Therapeutic Applications*, 60.

43 Ibid., 61–63.

patients suffering from sexually transmitted diseases.[44] Later on, these areas of applications were expanded: "Pillen I. Hals- und Brustleiden, Pillen II. und Wein Magen-, Leber-, Unterleibs-, und Hämorrhoidal-Beschwerden, Pillen III. und Spiritus Affectionen des Nervensystems, Neuralgien, Migraine, etc., allgemeine und spec. Schwächezustände jeder Art."[45] His colleague Dr Alvarez who worked an ocean away in Lima, Peru had products sold under his name by several German pharmacies. Dr Alvarez made a similar distinction between his pills but offered a fourth choice: "Die Pillen Nr. I eignen sich vorzüglich gegen die Leiden der Respirationsorgane, die Pillen Nr. II beseitigen alle Leiden der Verdauungsorgane, die Pillen Nr. III sind ein unfehlbares Heilmittel bei allen Nervenanomalien u. Schwächezuständen, die Pillen Nr. IV werden mit Erfolg bei Hämorrhoiden, starken Magenschmerzen etc. gebraucht."[46] Although both Dr Sampson and Dr Alavarez distinguished between three or four different kinds of pills, it was more a marketing strategy since the numbing and stimulating effects of coca could have produced relief in a majority of those complaints.

Coca products in Germany were significantly cheaper than those in Britain which greatly influenced their accessibility in both countries.[47] In Germany, pills such as those of Dr Sampson and Dr Alvarez were available in boxes of 100 and cost 1 Thaler each (3 Reichsmark after the monetary reform in 1871) or 5 Thaler (15 Reichsmark) for six which equalled about 8d.[48] The price for Alvarez' *coca spiritus* and *coca liqueur* was the same. Another coca liqueur such as that sold by a pharmacist in Düsseldorf cost a little less with 2 Reichsmark which was about 5d.[49] Those prices were consistent from the 1860s onwards but prices

44 "Lungenleiden, Schwächezustände," *Kölnische Zeitung* (2nd January 1870), 8.

45 "Prof. Dr. Sampson's Coca-Präparate," *Kölnische Zeitung* (3rd December 1873), 4.

46 "Coca-Präparate," *Bonner Zeitung* (8th November 1875), 4.

47 In subsequent paragraphs, the following monetary equivalents were taken as a basis: 90 Thaler (pre-1871) = 30 Reichsmark (post-1871) = £1 = 20 Shilling (s) = 240 pence (d). W A Shaw, *The History of Currency 1252 to 1894* (London: Clement Wilson, 1896), 215, 382, 393; "Money," University of Nottingham, accessed 18th June 2025, https://www.nottingham.ac.uk/manuscriptsandspecialcollections/researchguidance/weightsandmeasures/money.aspx.

48 "Asthma und Catarrhe der Luftwege," *Hannoverscher Kurier* (25th November 1878), 3; "Die wunderbaren Nähr- u. Heilkräfte...," *Rhein- und Ruhrzeitung* (30th September 1875), 4; "Coca Praeparate," *Bonner Zeitung* (8th November 1875), 4; "Schwächezustände alter und junger Männer...," *Kölnische Zeitung* (7th January 1867), 6.

49 "Aromatischen Coca-Liqueur," *Düsseldorfer Volksblatt* (24th April 1877), 6.

in Britain were still much higher in the 1890s, almost three decades after they had been introduced on the continent. Customers in Britain wanting to buy a bottle of British coca wine at the end of the century had to pay between 3s 6d and 3s 9d which was five to six times the German price.[50] On the one hand, this can be explained by Germany and France entering both the coca trade and coca research comparatively early which gave them a head start in the supply with coca leaves. On the other hand, the discrepancy in prices also evokes questions as to the actual coca content in those remedies.

In an article on coca published in the *Deutsche Apotheker-Zeitung* in 2016, Thomas Langebner argued that some of the coca pills contained iron powder and that German pharmacist Hermann Hager already objected the coca content in those products as early as 1876.[51] Given his professional expertise, Hager could test those products and concluded that they contained "hauptsächlich Stoffe, welche nicht Coca sind," which contributed to the "Cocaschwindel," a coca swindle.[52] If we remember the circumstances of the coca trade in Chapters I and II, it is easy to see that despite their early engagement, the procurement of sufficient and sufficiently potent leaves was still difficult and costly in the 1870s. The import lists for the port of Hamburg, which was the primary port of entrance for coca leaves, only listed them after 1885 and in Britain, they were first listed as a separate post in 1877. These imports and the analyses conducted by a German pharmacist give reason to believe that the actual amount of coca in German preparations was at least negligent, if not non-existent. The other way round, this reinforces the claim that British coca products were more authentic and actually *did* contain the active ingredient. This is supported by them being introduced into the British market much later and at a much higher price that made coca products only affordable for the upper middle and upper classes. As Bidie explained as late as 1885, "the only barriers to its [cocaine's, KE] extended use are its scarcity and costliness."[53]

A brief discussion surrounding the procurement of coca leaves in Britain emerged in the *British Medical Journal* when Dr E H Sieveking argued in Febru-

---

50 "Tonic Wine. Vinacoca Tonic Wine," *The Graphic* (18th October 1890), 28; "Armbrecht Coca Wine," *The Times* (24th February 1896), 13.

51 Thomas Langebner, "Über Coca in der westlichen Medizin," *Deutsche Apotheker-Zeitung*, last modified 4th June 2016, https://www.deutsche-apotheker-zeitung.de/news/artikel/2016/05/31/cocaine-coca-medical-use-pharmacopoeia-medizin/chapter:6.

52 Hermann Hager, *Handbuch der pharmaceutischen Praxis. Bd. 1* (Berlin: Springer, 1876), 905.

53 Bidie, *Coca, its Source, Culture, Uses, &c.*, 12.

ary 1874 that he was only able to obtain "a chest of coca leaves" from a private salesman and later from "Mr. Squire, her Majesty's chemist."[54] In successive issues of the journals, colleagues objected stating that "there has been no difficulty, for many years, in obtaining the leaves of this shrub in this country" and that apparently coca and preparations thereof, including cocaine, had been "for some years past been imported into this country from America."[55] J Alexander Bell even offered to supply fellow physicians with a small quantity should they desire to use it in their practice.[56] Others, such as William Carter from Liverpool received coca preparations from the Apothecaries' Company and Alexander Bennett, who investigated coca's physiological action reportedly acquired it "from various sources."[57] The accessibility of coca increased in the 1870s but it was still highly dependent on knowing the right people and places for acquisition.

As cocaine became known as a local anaesthetic in late 1884, the range of coca products was extended. The claim by some scientists, such as Hager, that the coca hype in Germany was little more than a hoax thus gained momentum again as the product range was priced comparatively low given the still highly irregular imports of coca and the costly purification process of cocaine at the time. It is likely, though, that the actual content of the drugs increased as availability increased and manufacturing costs decreased.

Merck of Darmstadt became the main producer of cocaine powder, first supplying only the European market but later expanding business to North America and beyond. Judging by German newspapers, the public was aware that the production of cocaine must have been very expensive but they seemed to have been ignorant of the actual price it was sold for. According to them, prices ranged from 8 Reichsmark to 129 Reichsmark per gram which exacerbated an average estimate.[58] Around the same time, the *British Medical Journal*

54 E H Sieveking, "Coca: Its Therapeutic Use," *British Medical Journal* (21st February 1874), 234.

55 Savory and Moore, "The Use of Coca," *British Medical Journal* (28th February 1874), 289; see also Arthur Leared, "The Use of Coca," *British Medical Journal* (28th February 1874), 272; J Alexander Bell, "The Use of Coca," *British Medical Journal* (7th March 1874), 305.

56 Bell, "The Use of Coca," 305.

57 William Carter, "The Use of Coca. IV," *British Medical Journal* (28th March 1874), 414; Bennett, "The Physiological Action of Coca," 510.

58 *Hannoverscher Kurier* (14th November 1884), 3; *Hannoverscher Kurier* (11th April 1885), 5; *Schwäbischer Merkur* (20th November 1884), 15; *Hallesches Tageblatt* (15th February 1885), 2; "(Ein neues Mittel gegen die Seekrankheit.)," *Hannoverscher Kurier* (18th November

spoke of 2s 6d for a grain (0.065g) and another magazine reported that the price in Britain dropped from £100 to £2 per ounce from 1885 to 1889.[59] If we apply the currency conversions used above, this meant a drop from around 320 to 6 Reichsmark per gram of cocaine in Germany which was an even higher price German newspapers gave in the early 1880s. Whatever the actual price was and despite it having varied from pharmacy to pharmacy, it can be agreed that cocaine was a luxurious narcotic that only the well-to-do could afford.

Due the high costs of manufacturing cocaine in Germany, pharmacists increasingly outsourced it to Peru where labourers produced crude cocaine in six different cities. Callao, a coastal city located next to Lima, exported 80% of the total amount.[60] Whereas this contributed to a decrease in cocaine prices in Europe, the production of coca leaves in Peru remained more profitable for them than the production of cocaine in the first years of the twentieth century. In 1906, for example, Peru produced over 3,223 t of coca valuing £130,325 as compared to 6.7 t of cocaine valuing £79,071 in the same year.[61] This outsourcing process caused the German pharmaceutical industry to continue research on cocaine which led to the discovery of ecgonine, another alkaloid of the coca plant but much less popular, and the creation of eucain hydrochlorate, a "synthetic cocain hydrochlorate."[62]

With increasing availability of both coca leaves and cocaine in Europe, the pharmaceutical industry in Germany and Britain used the range of coca products as a blueprint for cocaine products. Initially, cocaine was taken orally in a watery solution and must have produced a similar effect as coca wine since

---

1885), 6; "Cocain," *Hallesches Tageblatt* (19th December 1885), 4; "Die Herstellung des Cocains…," *Hallesches Tageblatt* (29th December 1885), 2; "Außerordentlich weit hat man es jetzt in der Anwendung schmerzstillender Mittel gebracht…," *Chemnitzer Anzeiger und Stadtbote* (14th March 1885), 2.

59 Crespi, "Some recent scientific Advances," 399; "Hydrochlorate of Cocaine, the new local Anaesthetic," *British Medical Journal* (29th November 1884), 1081; Mivart, "Cocaine," 1131; See also Bidie, *Coca, its Source, Culture, Uses, &c.*, 6, that stated prices per grain of cocaine between 2s 6d and 4s. Recall from Chapter II that an average British labourer earned about 25 shillings a week to feed his whole family, which equalled £1.25. The average salary for a German labourer was about 15 Reichsmark a week, 10 British shillings.

60 House of Commons, *Diplomatic and Consular Reports. Peru. Report for the Year 1907 on the Trade and Commerce of Peru* (London: Harrison and Sons, 1908), 30; The other five cities for cocaine production were Lima, Otuzco, Cajamarca, Huanta, and Cuzco.

61 House of Commons, *Report for the Year 1907*, 26.

62 "Eucain Hydrochlorate," Burroughs, Wellcome & Co, ca. 1896; "Die Herstellung des Cocains…," *Hallesches Tageblatt* (29th December 1885), 2.

the cocaine content in the solution amounted to only a few milligrams and was absorbed by tissue before it could unfold its full effect. Others, such as Mariani, simply added cocaine to some of their existing products to expand their product range. Surprisingly much less popular than *Vin Mariani*, *Pastilles Mariani* were the most potent drug in his assortment. Consisting of the same ingredients as the lozenges, 2 mg of pure cocaine were added to each lozenge and Mariani warned that "[t]heir action [was] much more intense and more rapid."[63] Those pastilles and cocaine in water thus had a similar effect while the former must have taken a little longer due to them being sucked rather than just swallowed. In American products, namely the famous Coca-Cola, cocaine was preferably mixed with non-alcoholic liquid and rapidly gained popularity as a stimulating beverage.[64]

The biggest manufacturer and wholesaler of cocaine products in Britain was Allen & Hanburys. By 1908, they offered no less than a dozen different products containing cocaine to various extents for a variety of purposes. Although they also carried coca wine – "Cokay" – and coca solutions, cocaine products were most profitable.[65] The cocaine content in those remedies ranged between 0,005 mg (ophthalmic lamels) and 5 g (Allenburys Solution Tablets) and depending on their mode of administration varied much in potency.[66] Although Allen & Hanburys had their own pharmacies, they also distributed their drugs to independent pharmacists who could buy them in dozens or thousands (pills) for wholesale prices. The cheapest product in their assortment were pessaries and suppositories which contained up to one gram of cocaine and started at 11d per dozen but given their application were probably the least popular.[67] At the other end of the spectrum were *Atomols*, atomizers, for as much as 1s a piece and *Azoules*, ampoules for hypodermic use, for 2s 6d per ten ampoules.[68]

63 Mariani, *Coca and its Therapeutic Applications*, 62.

64 The original Coca-Cola contained not only coca for flavour but also cocaine in an unknown amount. Although the US was more concerned about its caffeine content, chemical analyses in a lawsuit in 1915 concluded that there was no cocaine in the beverage which meant that it must have been removed from the recipe before then. Compare *US v. Forty Barrels and Twenty Kegs of Coca Cola*. 241 U.S. 265 (1915).

65 *General List of Drugs*, 165.

66 Ibid., 147, 148, 208.

67 *General List of Drugs*, 134.

68 Ibid., 184–186.

One of Allen & Hanbury's biggest competitors Burroughs, later also known as Burrough & Wellcome, offered a similar variety of products that included coca wine and coca solution, as well as cocaine voice, hypodermic, and compressed tabloids. Their tabloids cost 1s or 2s for two sizes of boxes and seemed very versatile in their applications as the company explained: "They may be employed either for ophthalmic, nasal, laryngeal, and endermic application as well as hypodermic injection."[69] Burroughs, Wellcome & Co also sold aluminium syringes for the hypodermic administration of cocaine but they were very expensive at 7s for one "with two regulation needles."[70]

Thanks to the Wellcome Foundation the secret recipe books of Burrough & Wellcome are now accessible to the wider public and reveal insightful details on the manufacturing of both coca and cocaine products. Although they date from 1913–1915, it can be assumed that those recipes had previously existed in some way before they were compromised in heavy and heavily secured volumes. As an unknown employee wrote in a statement: "The manufacture of cocaine started at the Wellcome Chemical Works as early as 1904 [...]."[71] This came comparatively late as Merck of Darmstadt had already manufactured cocaine for two decades at that time. However, Burrough and Wellcome became the second major cocaine producer in Britain after Allen & Hanbury which facilitated the availability and accessibility of the drug on the British market.

Whereas the actual content of coca leaf in final products was still questionable three decades prior – at least in a majority of products not tested by German pharmacist Hager – these recipe books unveiled the truth, at least for the years around 1913. In one recipe book, chemists explained how to manufacture their extract of coca liqueur and in another, they outlined the purification process of cocaine from coca leaves.[72] Whereas cocaine was usually used to be further processed as part of solutions or tablets in which the content varied,

69 "Cocaine "Tabloids."," leaflet, 27th November 1891, Burroughs, Wellcome & Co.

70 "The pure Aluminium hypodermic syringe," leaflet, ca. 1890s, Burroughs, Wellcome & Co.

71 "The Story of Cocaine," treatise, 27th February 1930, Wellcome Institute. This does not mean that Burroughs and Wellcome did not previously produce products with imported cocaine, though. Compare: W E to A Langman, 17th September 1903, letter, Wellcome Collection.

72 Chemical Department Burroughs Wellcome & Co, *Processes* (Book III), 1913; Chemical Department Burroughs Wellcome & Co, *Processes* (Book IV), 1913.

Burrough and Wellcome's extract of coca liqueur contained an astonishing 58% of coca.[73]

Another astonishing remark in the recipe books concerns the origin of the coca leaves used in the manufacturing process. As explained in Chapters I and II, coca did not grow in the British Empire to a significant extent to be used for domestic production which required the import of coca leaves of other origins. Burrough and Wellcome's recipe books stated in 1913 that "[f]inely crushed Java leaves were used" for the production of cocaine and they even "gave 1.29% total alkaloids" which was double the amount found in the British-grown Ceylon and Indian leaf in the 1880s.[74] However, in 1909, British officials stated that less than 1% of the Java leaf was exported to Britain.[75] This circumstance gives rise to the questions whether Java leaf was imported from other places, for example from Germany, or whether exports from Java to Britain increased in the years in between. The first explanation does not seem plausible as Germany primarily imported coca from South America as it was the best quality on the market and had done so for several decades. There was no need to import lower quality leaf from other far-away locations. It is more likely that the share of Java leaf exported to Britain increased due to higher demand which also eliminated the costs of stopovers at foreign ports.

At the turn of the century at the latest, consumers had plenty of choice of coca and cocaine products from different companies. Their quality improved significantly with more reliable supply chains of the drugs, both from overseas and by domestic manufacturing, and prices for these products dropped over time. Despite their outstanding medicinal properties and exceptional value for surgeries, many consumers were ignorant of the benefits of coca and cocaine which required pharmaceutical companies to raise awareness through advertising.

6. The Role of Advertising

Whereas the consumption of other narcotics, particularly that of opium, was so prevalent among British society that they did not need to be advertised for

73 100 lbs of coca leaves yielded 72 pints of liquid containing at least 40% alcohol.

74 Chemical Department Burroughs Wellcome & Co, *Processes* (Book III), 1913.

75 Compare Chapter II, "Excursus: The British-South Asian Axis."

the promotion of sales, coca entered the market as a novelty and therefore relied heavily on advertising. In fact, the advertisement of coca and later cocaine products was crucial for their career and flushed plenty of money into the pockets of the pharmaceutical industry.[76] This affected not only those who did research on the drug, but first and foremost the manufacturers and the apothecaries at the end of the line, so it was a win-win-situation for everyone involved. However, just like with any new product on the market, raising awareness for coca stood at the beginning of the process before branding, promotion, and reputation could determine its success or failure.

Pharmaceutical companies often tried different strategies to enlarge their consumer base, for example by handing out free samples or by advertising in a variety of newspapers at once and had to keep an eye on current medicinal developments that impacted the trajectory of coca products. This was especially relevant when negative consequences of coca's alkaloid cocaine became known and the line between medicinal and recreational consumption became blurred.

When coca products were first advertised, it was important to raise awareness for the existence of those products which also increased their visibility for potential customers. Unlike other exotic narcotics such as opium, which was well-known in Britain, many people had never heard of the "divine plant of the Incas" and therefore had to learn about its origin and effects first.[77] The circumstance of various newspapers previously reporting about the habit of coca chewing in South America, the *Novara* expedition, and Niemann was conducive for coca advertising in Germany because the regular reader would have known at least a little bit about its discovery before coca products entered the pharmaceutical market. Subsequently, these reports were also highly influential for the success of coca products because journalists would write about their benefits and cover news about coca research. In Britain, however, such reports did not make it into public newspapers until coca products were already popular on the continent. Consequently, British consumer lacked knowledge about coca in comparison to Germans, thus hampering the number of sales which did not increase as rapidly on the island.

Dr Sampson's coca pills were one of the first coca products that were advertised in German newspapers in the early 1860s and pharmacies offered free

76 Gootenberg, *Andean Cocaine*, 57.

77 Mortimer, *History of Coca*, 227.

brochures containing information on the coca plant and its effects.[78] Later on, these adverts also contained references from famous explorers in South America, for example Alexander von Humboldt, Herman von Boerhaave, and Tschudi, that drew the public's attention to coca and fostered the credibility of its medicinal value.[79] In Britain, adverts such as those for *Vin Mariani* regularly appeared in a couple of newspapers but they only occurred after the 1880s and were characterised by an absence of such references. Britain did not have any explorers who could lend credence to coca and it is questionable whether references to German or Dutch explorers would have proved a good selling point there.

From the very beginning when coca was rediscovered and introduced into the European market, Germany managed to advertise coca products better than Britain which significantly influenced public awareness of coca products across the country. In the 1860s, coca adverts appeared in a handful of newspaper titles about every three weeks but this increased up to twice a week in the mid-1870s. In contrast to that, visibility of coca adverts in British newspapers was very limited. Market leader Mariani seemed to have been the only one who regularly advertised his *Vin* and it was not until the 1890s that other products like *Vinacoca* and Lorimer's coca wine made a regular appearance in *The Times, The Daily News, The Era*, the *Pall Mall Gazette*, and others. This development happened relatively late when coca was almost outdated in Germany due to the fascination with cocaine.

Besides of coca adverts in print media, the British pharmaceutical industry also resorted to giving out leaflets and informative papers in apothecaries. This improved credibility and gave pharmaceutical companies the opportunity to explain the origins and benefits of their coca products in depth. Leaflets were the favoured mode of advertising for Hall's, (James) Burrough's, Burrough & Wellcome's, and Home's coca wine. It posed an alternative way of advertising and appealed to a broader consumer base as they were free and did not require a newspaper or journal to be bought to access information about a new drug on the market. As historian Simon Cooke put it,

---

78 "Dr. medic. Samson's Coca-Pillen," *Echo der Gegenwart* (13th March 1867), 3; "Lungenleiden, Schwächezustände," *Kölnische Zeitung* (2nd January 1870), 8.

79 "Coca-Pillen I, II & III," *Echo der Gegenwart* (14th April 1872), 3; "Die wunderbaren Nähr- u. Heilkräfte...," *Rhein- und Ruhrzeitung*, 4.

> [...] [M]ost Victorian advertisers sought to promote their wares not through the agency of slogans, but by trying to persuade the consumer to buy by explaining the qualities of their product at great length, and sometimes in microscopic detail. This laborious over-writing seems to have been equated in the public mind with authority: the more that was written, and the greater the elaboration, the greater the likelihood of the product's and seller's integrity.[80]

Those leaflets primarily appealed to upper-class citizens shopping in pharmacies which expanded the reach of coca advertising.

Coca adverts for a specific product were usually consistent and printed across different newspapers and journals which facilitated the work of advertisers and made the product easier to recognise for customers. Special features such as characteristic drawings, font, repetitions, and size made the adverts memorable and contributed to brand recognition. The most popular feature was certainly repetition which increased visibility on a huge newspaper page that was full of adverts for other products and services. Just compare the three adverts on the next page for *Vin Mariani*, Lorimer's Coca Wine, and Jesse William's Coca Wine (Fig. 1–3) and imagine them on a black and white DIN A2 page. Other adverts, such as those for Dr Alvarez' coca pills, Dr Sampson's coca pills, and *Vinacoca* (Fig. 4, 5, 7) resorted to unique embellishments like banderoles, coca leaf shapes, or a coca leaf twig that made them stand out. In contrast to the other coca products mentioned, Armbrecht occasionally decided to make an impact by size and advertised his coca wine on the whole left side of a page of *The Times* (Fig. 6).[81] This gave the company the opportunity to explain the active principles, medicinal value, range of applications, and alternative products in his assortment similar to leaflets, but it is questionable whether readers made an effort to read through the whole advert. It is likely, though, that they took advantage of his offer to obtain a free bottle of coca wine to judge for themselves.[82]

---

80 Simon Cooke, "Advertisements in Victorian Books and Magazines," The Victorian Web, last amended 25th July 2019, https://victorianweb.org/victorian/art/design/advertisements/cooke.html.

81 "Armbrecht Coca Wine," *The Times*, 13. Due to its size, it will not be reprinted here in full.

82 Stephen Smith & Co similarly offered free samples of Hall's coca wine, see "Free Test," *Longman's Magazine* (April 1897), 29.

Figure 1: Top part of advert for Vin Mariani.

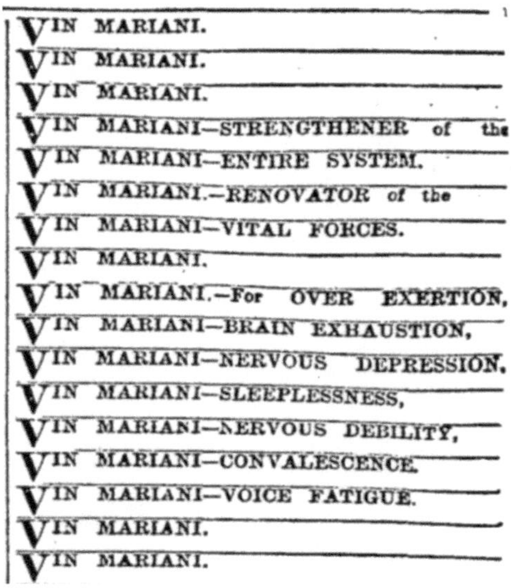

The Times (27th September 1892), 10.

Figure 2: Advert for Jesse Williams's Coca Wine.

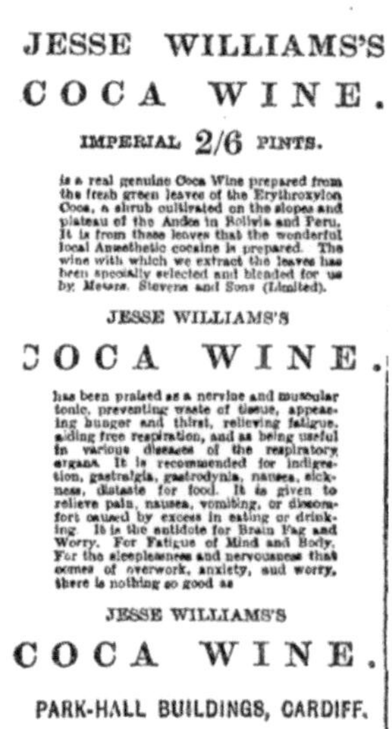
JESSE WILLIAMS'S
COCA WINE.
IMPERIAL 2/6 PINTS.
is a real genuine Coca Wine prepared from the fresh green leaves of the Erythroxylon Coca, a shrub cultivated on the slopes and plateau of the Andes in Bolivia and Peru. It is from these leaves that the wonderful local Anaesthetic cocaine is prepared. The wine with which we extract the leaves has been specially selected and blended for us by Messrs. Stevens and Sons (Limited).
JESSE WILLIAMS'S
COCA WINE.
has been praised as a nervine and muscular tonic, preventing waste of tissue, appeasing hunger and thirst, relieving fatigue, aiding free respiration, and as being useful in various diseases of the respiratory organs. It is recommended for indigestion, gastralgia, gastrodynia, nausea, sickness, distaste for food. It is given to relieve pain, nausea, vomiting, or discomfort caused by excess in eating or drinking. It is the antidote for Brain Fag and Worry. For Fatigue of Mind and Body. For the sleeplessness and nervousness that comes of overwork, anxiety, and worry, there is nothing so good as
JESSE WILLIAMS'S
COCA WINE.
PARK-HALL BUILDINGS, CARDIFF.

Western Mail (5th January 1897), 3.

Figure 3: Advert for Lorimer's Coca Wine.

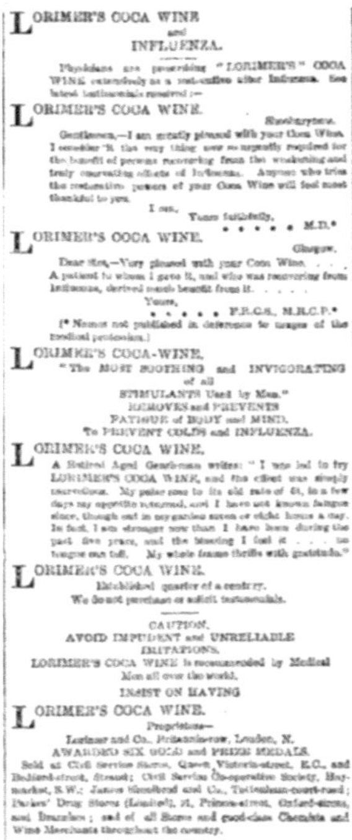
LORIMER'S COCA WINE
and
INFLUENZA.
LORIMER'S COCA WINE.
LORIMER'S COCA WINE.
LORIMER'S COCA-WINE.
"The MOST SOOTHING and INVIGORATING
of all
STIMULANTS Used by Man."
REMOVES and PREVENTS
FATIGUE of BODY and MIND.
To PREVENT COLDS and INFLUENZA.
LORIMER'S COCA WINE.
LORIMER'S COCA WINE.
CAUTION.
AVOID IMPUDENT and UNRELIABLE
IMITATIONS.
LORIMER'S COCA WINE is recommended by Medical
Men all over the world.
INSIST ON HAVING
LORIMER'S COCA WINE.
AWARDED SIX GOLD and PRIZE MEDALS.

The Daily News (28th February 1895), 4.

Figure 4: Advert for Vinacoca Tonic Wine.

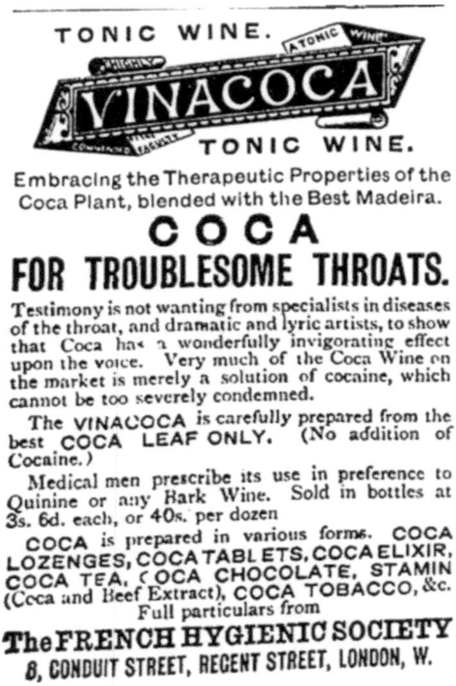
TONIC WINE.
A TONIC WINE
VINACOCA
TONIC WINE.
Embracing the Therapeutic Properties of the
Coca Plant, blended with the Best Madeira.
COCA
FOR TROUBLESOME THROATS.
Testimony is not wanting from specialists in diseases of the throat, and dramatic and lyric artists, to show that Coca has a wonderfully invigorating effect upon the voice. Very much of the Coca Wine on the market is merely a solution of cocaine, which cannot be too severely condemned.
The VINACOCA is carefully prepared from the best COCA LEAF ONLY. (No addition of Cocaine.)
Medical men prescribe its use in preference to Quinine or any Bark Wine. Sold in bottles at 3s. 6d. each, or 40s. per dozen
COCA is prepared in various forms. COCA LOZENGES, COCA TABLETS, COCA ELIXIR, COCA TEA, COCA CHOCOLATE, STAMIN (Coca and Beef Extract), COCA TOBACCO, &c.
Full particulars from
The FRENCH HYGIENIC SOCIETY
8, CONDUIT STREET, REGENT STREET, LONDON, W.

The Graphic (18th October 1890), 28.

Figure 5: Advert for Dr Alvarez' Coca Preparations.

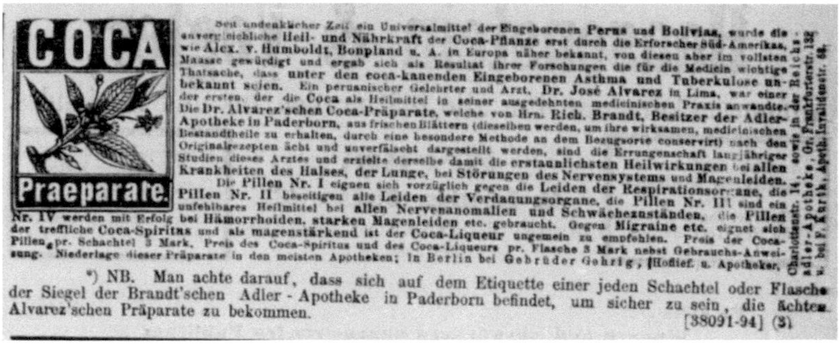

Berliner Börsen-Zeitung (28th November 1875), 15.

Figure 6: Top part of an advert for Armbrecht's Coca Wine.

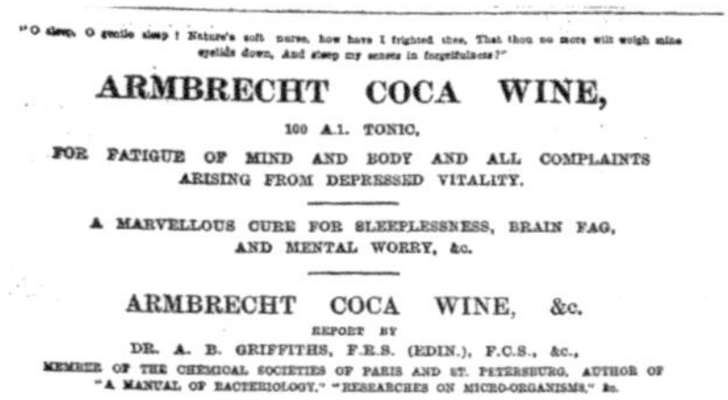

The Times (24th February 1896), 13.

Figure 7: Advert for Prof Dr Sampson's Coca Preparations.

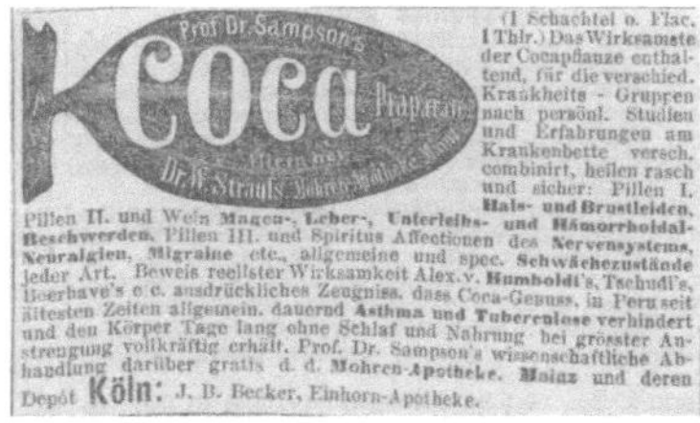
Prof Dr Sampson's
Coca
(1 Schachtel o. Flac. 1 Thlr.) Das Wirksamste der Cocapflanze enthaltend, für die verschied. Krankheits-Gruppen nach persönl. Studien und Erfahrungen am Krankenbette versch. combinirt, heilen rasch und sicher: Pillen I. Hals- und Brustleiden, Pillen II. und Wein Magen-, Leber-, Unterleibs- und Hämorrhoidal-Beschwerden, Pillen III. und Spiritus Affectionen des Nervensystems, Neuralgien, Migraine etc., allgemeine und spec. Schwächezustände jeder Art. Beweis reellster Wirksamkeit Alex. v. Humboldt's, Tschudi's, Boerhave's etc. ausdrückliches Zeugniss, dass Coca-Genuss, in Peru seit ältesten Zeiten allgemein, dauernd Asthma und Tuberculose verhindert und den Körper Tage lang ohne Schlaf und Nahrung bei grösster Anstrengung vollkräftig erhält. Prof. Dr. Sampson's wissenschaftliche Abhandlung darüber gratis d. d. Mohren-Apotheke, Mainz und deren Depôt Köln: J. B. Becker, Einhorn-Apotheke.

Kölnische Zeitung (3rd December 1873), 4

Apart from free product samples, which posed an exception in coca advertising, consumer perception was primarily shaped by highlighting the drug's exoticism and its value against a variety of ailments. References to explorers created the impression that consumers could partake in their ventures by obtaining a product that originated in a faraway country outside the British Empire. Opium, as the prominent vanguard in narcotics, for example, was not considered as exotic anymore and could therefore not resort to that being an exceptional feature to boost sales. Cannabis as another example and narcotic being on the rise in the late-nineteenth century was mainly grown in India which made it an imperial product and similarly deducted from its exoticism.[83] The fascination with the primitive that I explain in detail in a later chapter, proved a unique selling point for coca products and was usually an integral part of adverts.

Besides coca's unique exotic origins, manufacturers also emphasised coca's outstanding properties to battle respiratory and gastrointestinal illnesses. As one German newspaper stated: "Keine Pflanze des Erdballs vereinigt so glücklich die heilsamsten Wirkungen auf die gesammten Organe der Athmung und Verdauung mit so enormer, konstanter Kräftigung des ganzen Nerven- und Muskelsystems als das Universalheilmittel der Indianer."[84] Coca's field of application was more limited than that of the all-time panacea opium but at the same time, this made applications more effective because they were better tailored to patients' needs. As Stephen Smith & Co explained in one of their leaflets; "Hall's coca wine is not a patent medicine. It does not claim to cure "all the ills the flesh is heir to"."[85] Coca was not a one-size-fits-all but it was a much better remedy for specific illnesses where opium could have merely alleviated side effects instead of fighting the cause itself.[86]

---

83 House of Commons, *Statement exhibiting the Moral and Material Progress and Condition of India during the Year 1870–71* (London: Eyre and Spottiswoode, 1872), 17; House of Commons, *Statement exhibiting the Moral and Material Progress and Condition of India during the Year 1874–75* (London: Eyre and Spottiswoode, 1876), 18; House of Commons. *Report on the Indian Excise Committee 1905–06* (London: Darling & Sons, 1907), 2.

84 "Coca-Pillen I, II & III," *Echo der Gegenwart*, 3, transl.: "No plant on this planet unifies so superbly the most salutary effects on all respiratory and intestinal organs with such tremendous and consistent invigoration of the whole neuronal and muscular system than the universal remedy of the Indians."

85 "Hall's Coca Wine," leaflet, no 194: 14, Wellcome Collection.

86 Ineffectiveness of many pain-relieving remedies which did not remove the cause was also mentioned in "Some Popular Remedies," *Chamber's Journal* (19th January 1895), 45.

Apart from its value in pulmonology and gastroenterology, coca also stood out as a stimulating tonic. Although it prevented fatigue similarly like caffeinated beverages such as coffee and tea, it produced a more exhilarating effect and could sustain hunger at the same time. This effect was reinforced with the arrival of the more potent cocaine. Cocaine was therefore thought to be helpful in mental illnesses where sedatives like opium and morphine would have produced a counterproductive effect. As a result, cocaine was occasionally advertised as a remedy not only against depressions but also as a remedy against opium and morphine addiction.[87] Wrote Burroughs & Wellcome: "Cocaine is antagonistic to opium, and has cured morphino-mania and alcoholic craving."[88] Sadly, this often led to a patient suffering from two addictions instead of one and it caused them to find themselves in a worse state of health than before. This development in the 1890s led to advertisements of rehabilitation centres such as that of the Keeley Institutes in Denmark.[89] For the pharmaceutical sector, including manufacturers and chemists in apothecaries, this was a win-win situation: First, they made money selling the drugs, then they made more money helping people getting away from them. At the end it was always the consumer who suffered, at least financially, but most definitely from a health perspective.

Adverts in British print media for rehab centres were still scarce and they did not have a significant impact on sales of coca and cocaine products. As pointed out above, those products were not affordable for the lower classes and even regular use, or abuse, would have been very costly so that cocaine addiction must not have been very prevalent. It is more probable that those institutes included cocaine as a new potentially harmful narcotic that was added to the list. Cures for narcotic addiction, especially morphinism, and alcoholism primarily targeted the upper classes who could afford it and were desperate enough to seek treatment on the continent.

Although not as extensive as in German print media, avid readers regularly came across adverts that appeared weekly or bi-weekly in renown newspapers such as the *Times*, the *Western Mail*, the *Daily News*, the *Era*, the *Graphic*, and the *Pall Mall Gazette*. Other magazines and journals included the *Academy*, the

87 Sigmund Freud became a prominent advocator of this.

88 "Hypodermic medication. Notes on Alkaloids. Antidote Tables and Precautions," miniature booklet, ca. 1890s, Burroughs & Wellcome, 6.

89 "Drunkenness, Morphine, Opium & Cocaine Habits," *The Daily News* (28th March 1893), 11.

Examiner, and *Chamber's Journal*. The dissemination of adverts in all these titles appealed to the middle and upper classes' curiosity of those drugs which increased popularity and sales. Apart from advertising in print media, everyone entering a pharmacy in Britain also had access to leaflets on cocaine products which were free and caught the eye of the potential customer. Those customers who required regular medical attendance or had long-lasting illnesses that made them a familiar face in the pharmacy certainly came across those leaflets and could foster word-of-mouth recommendation. Only a few adverts for rehabs and negative reports on narcotics were published in public media.

As the British pharmaceutical market offered coca wine and cocaine pills from a variety of companies, it was essential for them to properly position their products on the market to distinguish them from those of competitors. One strategy to highlight the uniqueness of a specific coca wine was to emphasise that it was the real deal, i.e., that it actually contained coca leaves and did not have any cocaine added. Especially in Germany, as previously explained, this was not self-evident and even in Britain, Mariani warned that "there [we]re several Fraudulent and Worthless Imitations of this valuable preparations."[90] Armbrecht sounded a similar note of caution stating that "[i]f you wish for good results, don't take imitations […]."[91] Contrary to their possible marketing strategy to lure customers into buying the brand product, the difficult and costly procurement and manufacturing of coca leaves rather contributed to a higher quality of the products of better known pharmaceutical companies. The French Hygienic Society ensured that their *Vinacoca* was "carefully prepared from the best COCA LEAF ONLY. (No addition of Cocaine.)."[92]

Another strategy to single out one's product and to prevent fraud was an easily recognisable design. Copycats of popular brands were also found for coca products which caused companies to resort to stand-alone features. Mariani regularly issued words of caution to only buy his *Vin* in bottles that show its name on the outside wrap, and Burrough's coca wine was known as the 'Red Cross Brand' as it showed a big red cross on the front of the bottles.[93] Stephen Smith & Co recommended "to insist on having 'HALL'S,' and seeing that the red

90 "Fraud. Important Notice. Vin Mariani-Coca Wine," *The Era* (5th May 1883), 2.

91 "Armbrecht Coca Wine," *The Times*, 13.

92 "Vinacoca," *The Graphic* (18th October 1890), 28.

93 Mariani, *Coca and its Therapeutic Applications*, 78; "James Burrough's Coca Wine," leaflet, ca. 1890s, Wellcome Collection.

'Keystone' Trade Mark is on every package."[94] Although quackery was first and foremost a problem before the introduction of the Pharmacy Act 1868, there were also non-licensed sellers who did not only copy popular brands but sold medicine that did not even contain the promised drug.[95]

Once pharmaceutical companies had their products on the market and ensured that they were well advertised, they needed to gain and maintain the public's trust through a favourable reputation. One pharmacist who became a pioneer in advertising medicine and whose prominence therefore endured the times by growing in popularity not only in his home country but also overseas was Mariani. From the moment he advertised his famous *Vin*, he realised that he had to rely on professional opinion to support his brand. Unbeknownst to the public, Mariani's close friend Dr Charles Fauvel, a laryngologist, became a fervent advocator for his products and benefitted from prescribing them to his patients. Other physicians both in continental Europe and Britain such as Dr Morell Mackenzie soon followed in assuring their support.[96] The Mariani brand also established his reputation in continental Europe and North America with prominent supporters such as world theatre star Sarah Bernhardt, Pope Leo XIII and US president Ulysses S Grant.[97]

Those important figures made it difficult for any of Mariani's competitors to catch up and they often resorted to claims that their products were supported by the medical profession, medical men, or the medical world. Some bigger pharmaceutical companies, like Burroughs, Wellcome & Co and Stephen & Smith Co could resort to actual physicians as testimonials who contributed to the public's trust in their brands. Dr A B Griffiths, for example, confirmed that "Burrough's Coca Wine [was] second to no other Coca Wine on the market" and Dr Peel Richards claimed that Hall's coca wine was "the first Coca Wine [he had] met with deserving the name."[98] Armbrecht decided on a somewhat different strategy in having Sir Christison and Sir Clements Markham confirm the marvellous effect of the most important ingredient in the products, coca.[99] In any way, those prominent professional supporters

94 "Hall's Wine," leaflet, ca. 1890, Wellcome Collection.

95 Holloway, *Royal Pharmaceutical Society of Great Britain, 1841–1991*, 224.

96 Mariani, *Coca and its Therapeutic Applications*, 55.

97 "Vin Mariani," *All the year round* (15th August 1891), 6.

98 "Burrough Coca Wine Chelsea Erythroxylon Coca," leaflet, ca. 1896, Wellcome Collection; "Hall's Coca Wine is not a patent medicine," leaflet, ca. 1890s, Wellcome Collection.

99 "Armbrecht Coca Wine," *The Times*, 13.

greatly contributed to establish well-known brands that gained the public's trust in the effectiveness of their coca products.

This similarly applied to cocaine products. Although British consuls thought the German pharmaceutical industry was "overdone and overrun" and objected that new products were not "properly tried" before their introduction to the market, German cocaine products became very popular and gained some well-known supporters, such as Sigmund Freud.[100] Freud was an Austrian psychiatrist, who later became known as the father of psychoanalysis, and who contributed to the popularity of cocaine in German-speaking countries. In his famous essay "Ueber Coca," Freud explained his experiments with cocaine on himself, consuming 0,05g cocaine in a watery solution about a dozen times.[101] He concluded that coca was indeed a valuable medicine that could be applied as a stimulant, against gastroenteric ailments, cachexia, and asthma, as well as to a smaller extent as an antidote against opium addiction and as an anaesthetic.[102] Nevertheless, Freud's essay did not spark sufficient curiosity in the medical community as it lacked closer scientific analysis wherefore his colleague and friend Koller carried off the laurels.

Due to continuous advertising efforts both in British and continental print media, coca products, and particularly coca wine, remained a sought-after product even when cocaine surpassed the original plant's potency and expanded medical application. They were reliable remedies, comparatively safe and much more affordable than the new marvel on the market which primarily drew its marvelousness from its expensive hypodermic application. Nevertheless, innovation in coca medicine was limited whereas constant innovations appeared in cocaine medicine: its initial discovery, watery solutions for local anaesthesia, solutions as a reviving tonic, and eventually hypodermic and intravenous administration. Although coca medicine had been popular for decades even with the co-existence of cocaine medicine, the latter had the upper hand in the first years of the twentieth century.

Coca products in Britain gained popularity at a time when the much more potent cocaine acted as a juggernaut for the pharmaceutical industry in Germany. This once again set the career of coca in Britain back. Not only did Germany have a head start with the earlier commencement of trade with

100 House of Commons, *Diplomatic and Consular Reports on Trade and Finance. Germany. Report for the Year 1895 on the Trade of Mannheim* (London: Harrison and Sons, 1896), 8.

101 Freud, "Ueber Coca," 299, 301.

102 Ibid., 304–314.

South America, but its researchers Niemann and Koller also pushed further and helped boost the cocaine industry that Britain could not catch up with. Whereas historian Paul Gootenberg acknowledged Germany becoming the "principal locus of world research, production, and distribution" of cocaine, he contradicted the first argument in stating that there was no real competition between the countries. [103] It was just that "Germans admired cocaine and the French and British preferred coca [...]."[104] However, this claim is too short-sighted. As previously explained, Britain plainly lacked the means to make cocaine more popular there due to irregular supply of the raw material and high costs of transport, manufacturing, and sales. Consequently, the consumer base for cocaine and possibilities to expand the market in Britain were limited.

Cocaine advocator Freud claimed that coca products had not experienced as much curiosity and popularity in Europe in general as in North America. He argued that the "ungünstige Erfolge, von denen bald nach der Einführung der Coca in Europa berichtet wurde, die zweifelhafte Güte, die Seltenheit und der hohe Preis der Präparate" greatly contributed to that, albeit undeservedly so.[105] He was right that both coca and cocaine became popular in the US more rapidly which led to other problems in that country but he did not make a distinction between coca and cocaine products. Coca products did in fact enjoy popularity in Europe but it was cocaine that was out of reach for most people in the late-nineteenth century.

The trajectory of coca in Britain in the Victorian Era thus highly depended on three key factors: availability, accessibility, and affordability. These were supported by clever advertising. Availability concerned the presence of coca products in pharmacies and them being prescribed by physicians. By the end of the century, customers could obtain them from at least the bigger pharmacies across the country and could even have them imported from the continent upon request. This facilitated accessibility which was also enabled by easy modes of consumption. Patients did not necessarily have to go to practices to have the drug administered but they could buy wines, lozenges, and tabloids for safe use at home without a prescription. The only limiting factor was

103 Gootenberg, *Andean Cocaine*, 26.

104 Ibid., 57.

105 Freud, "Ueber Coca," 304, transl.: "unfavourable successes that were reported soon after the introduction of coca in Europe, the questionable quality, the rarity, and the high price of the preparations."

affordability due to procurement and manufacturing costs, particularly with the arrival of cocaine. Whereas coca products were still somewhat affordable for the middle classes, cocaine products were destined for the upper classes. Prices for cocaine dropped around the turn of the century but supplies for hypodermic application such as syringes were still high which did not necessarily decrease the costs in total. Although advertisement could influence the availability and accessibility to a certain extent, it could not influence the trajectory of coca in terms of affordability. Still, it played a crucial role for the pharmaceutical industry.

7. Crossing the Line

Coca products experienced its heyday between the 1860s and 1880s, primarily in France and Germany. After the arrival of cocaine in the 1880s, the pharmaceutical landscape changed to a certain extent as the original plant yielded a far more potent alkaloid that could be applied in different ways to revolutionise anaesthesia. But with those extended possibilities also came increased risks. The medical and pharmaceutical professions grew increasingly aware of consequences of regular (increasing) use of coca and cocaine that spared no-one and could become a danger to public health. As a result, many products were warned of but instead of going after the marvellous but dangerous cocaine first, they aimed at the rather innocuous coca.

The debate about the dangers emanating from coca wines primarily emerged from them not being patent medicine and thus not being controlled by the state. Unlike laudanum and other opium preparations that were required to have a set narcotic content and follow a recipe, coca wines were not regulated. The amount of the narcotic agent was therefore volatile and customers purchasing coca wine from different brands and pharmacies either experienced weaker or stronger effects than what they had been used to. This was especially true once cocaine was added to some coca wines which significantly boosted its potency. On the one hand, this volatility increased competition between manufacturers but the lack of transparency upset customers and called for regulative action. The pharmaceutical industry did not react to this development in a timely and adequate manner which led to potentially harmless and medicinally beneficial coca wines to be vilified.

It is therefore not surprising that alleged market leaders such as Mariani regularly reassured customers in their adverts that their coca wine only contained coca leaves or extract thereof and not the pure alkaloid. However, this did not prevent the spread of critical voices since several copycats still added cocaine to their coca wines. As the *British Medical Journal* stated in 1897, "[o]riginally coca wine was made from coca leaves, but it is now commonly a solution of the alkaloid in a sweet and usually strongly alcoholic wine."[106] Despite the lack of a 'purity law' for coca wines, producers adding cocaine and not declaring it, which significantly increased their potency, exacerbated a medical verdict on coca wines in general.[107] As a result, it got increasing difficult for coca manufacturers to promote their products in this atmosphere. In France, for example, *Vin Mariani* was taken off the French Pharmaceutical Index in 1910 because it was considered detrimental to public health. It did not take long until Britain also jumped on the bandwagon in disparaging coca wines as it seemed easier to ban both coca and cocaine than to make a reasonable decision based on actual contents in products.

The challenge to assess the risk of coca products on the market thus stemmed from the difficulty of not knowing the exact amount of the active principles in the remedies and from a lack of scientific data to back up knowledge of potentially dangerous amounts. As established prior, coca leaves contain only about 0.5% cocaine and despite their good solvability in alcohol, such beverages do not by far have the same effect as pure cocaine in alcohol. Still, coca and cocaine were often used synonymously which contradicted their actual effects on the human body. The mode of application also played a rather negligible role. Nevertheless, a few physicians rightfully highlighted that the drugs' action varied in consumers which complicated the determination of risky amounts: "Cocaine may be toxic, sometimes deadly, in large doses. It may give rise to dangerous, or even fatal, symptoms in doses usually deemed safe. The danger, near and remote, is greatest when given under the skin."[108]

Of primary concern for the medical profession were women and children whose ignorance would lead them into an addiction not only of the narcotic but of alcohol as well.[109] The concern for women becoming alcohol addicts

106 "Coca Wine and its Salts," *British Medical Journal* (6th February 1897), 353.

107 Compare "The Dangers of Coca Wines." *British Medical Journal* (4th December 1897), 1666 and Frederic C Coley, "Medicated Wines," *British Medical Journal* (10th September 1898), 716.

108 Mattison, "Cocaine Dosage and Cocaine Addiction," 1026.

109 Coley, "Medicated Wines," 716; "The Dangers of Coca Wines," *British Medical Journal* (4th December 1897), 1666.

was not new, as it was not deemed appropriate for them to indulge in such morally questionable habits. The concern for children, however, was relatively new as generations of Victorian children, particularly of the working class, were drugged with opium in their young lives. Back then, this was both a necessity, as other pain relief was more expensive, and a burden since parents risked overdosing and addiction.[110] So, when it came to coca wine at the end of the nineteenth century, it was argued that children would become addicted to both coca – or cocaine, depending on the coca wine – and alcohol which needed to be prevented. This development reflected a heightened awareness of the concept of addiction that affected the most vulnerable members of society.

From a modern point of view, it is surprising that physicians and pharmacists worried about coca preparations the same way they worried about hypodermic applications of cocaine. Still, this illustrated an increasing awareness for the health risks of narcotics at the turn of the century. Voices of cocainism following morphinomania grew louder which made the medical and pharmaceutical profession overly cautious towards new narcotic products on the market, regardless of their mode of application.[111] At the same time, the concept of addiction as an illness emerged and made people realise that there was more to narcotic consumption that it merely being a habit or a vice.

Historian Virginia Berridge has claimed that the conviction of addiction being a medical condition that needed to be treated only evolved after the mid-nineteenth century in conjunction with the development of the disease theory and the greater involvement of the medical profession with hypodermic applications.[112] Although she highlighted that hypodermic administration of narcotics differed in the mode of consumption from opium and contributed greatly to the concept of addiction, she failed to explain why less dangerous drugs such as coca were painted with the same brush.[113]

Indeed, as late as the 1890s, the *British Medical Journal* increased awareness for the dangers emanating from coca wines when actually, cocaine injections should have been much more reason for concern.[114] The reason lied in the

110 Berridge and Edwards, *Opium and the People*, 98, 99, 102.

111 Mattison, "Cocaine Dosage and Cocaine Addiction," 1024–1026.

112 Berridge, "Morality and Medical Science," 67.

113 Ibid., 75.

114 "Coca Wine and Its Dangers," *British Medical Journal* (6th February 1897), 353; "The Dangers of Coca Wines," *British Medical Journal*, 1666.

broader debate of narcotics and addiction at the time that was less concerned with them becoming a danger to individual health but more with them becoming a threat to the health of society as a whole.

Not neglectable and rather indispensable for the pharmaceutical industry in this context was the rise of recreational use of coca and especially of cocaine during the last decade of the nineteenth century. Given their medicinal and at the same time stimulative properties, it was not surprising that the line between medicinal and recreational use became blurred. Often patients started off with having these narcotics prescribed from a physician, or consumers bought them for specific ailments from the local pharmacy. Others sought to break off an opium or morphine habit but this was often considered a transitionary phase to chronic cocaine consumption.[115] At the beginning it might have helped the cause but upon withdrawal, consumers realised their stimulating effect which was difficult to abandon when there was no medical indication anymore. This continuance of consumption formed a habit, and Victorians only slowly understood this as addiction, as an illness that had to be treated.

The trajectory of coca as a valuable novel narcotic that turned into a vicious vice was thus the result of increasing medicalisation.[116] Looking at coca and cocaine consumption discussed in this chapter, it is obvious that various actors and actions contributed to the pathologization of what was initially considered merely a 'moral failing' or 'weakness of character.' These included medical professionals, consumers, and bystanders as actors, but also new evidence about the effects of narcotics on the human body and new treatments against narcotic dependence. Eventually, this medicalisation propelled stricter drug regulations such as the Pharmacy Act 1868 that is explained in Chapter V.

---

115 This was also echoed in German newspapers: "[...] hier [lag] der Uebergang zum chronischen Cocainismus, zum letzen Modelaster," transl.: "[...] herein lies the transition to chronic cocainism, to the latest vice," "Locales. Die Gefährlichkeit mancher modernen Heilmittel...," *Berliner Börsen-Zeitung* (20th August 1889), 5.

116 As sociologists Peter Conrad and Kristin K Barker observed: "Medicalization occurs when human problems or experiences become defined as medical problems, usually in terms of illnesses, diseases, or syndromes" which emphasises "the processes by which a particular diagnosis is developed, becomes accepted as medically valid, and gets used to define and treat patients' problems," see Peter Conrad and Kristin K Barker, "The Social Construction of Illness: Key Insights and Policy Implications," *Journal of Health and Social Behavior* Volume 51, Issue 1 (2010), 74.

However, there remains some dissonance about the medicalisation of coca in comparison to other narcotics such as opium and morphine. Between the introduction of the first coca products on the market in the 1860s and the publication of adverts for rehab centres only twenty years passed, yet opium that had been used for over a century before encountering similar opposition. This raises the question as to why coca and cocaine faced such a rapid medicalisation. The answer lies not specifically in medicalisation but in the overarching scientification that took place during the last decades of the nineteenth century.

The scientification of society was visible in a broader reliance on empirical research, professional expertise, and systemic approaches to problems concerning public health which posed a rejection of primarily moral considerations.[117] The chemical analysis of narcotics allowed for a better understanding of their physiological effects which was then disseminated in medical journals and societies as a topic of scientific enquiry. In addition, medical education became more standardised after the foundation of institutions such as the Royal Pharmaceutical Society and highlighted the importance of scientific principles in medical practice. This became especially relevant with the discovery of more potent narcotics and the arrival of new medical equipment, particularly the hypodermic syringe. Moreover, as public health emerged as a subdiscipline, debates surrounding narcotic consumption blended previous moral concerns with scientific findings and eventually fuelled social reform movements, such as the temperance movement. I discuss the sociocultural aspects in more detail in the following chapter.

The awareness of the problem that excessive cocaine consumption posed to Victorian society thus stemmed from the evolution of medicalisation that was deeply tied to scientification in the same era. Coca did not experience a short-lived career from its introduction on the British market to international regulations because of its individual characteristics but because it was one of several narcotics that faced the same fate, regardless of how long they had been in use.

---

117 For a general explanation of scientification of society see Hubert Knoblauch, "Reflexive Methodology and the Empirical Theory of Science," *Historical Social Research / Historische Sozialforschung* 46, no. 2 (2021), 61, 62.

Chapter IV: Coca as Crowd-Pleaser?!

1. Cultural Dissimilation

It was not until medicinal and economic circumstances facilitated the introduction of a novel narcotic on the market that sociocultural currents both accelerated and exacerbated coca's career. Before the medicinal benefits or risks of coca became known, it was difficult for society to form an educated opinion, especially since clever advertising of coca products made it challenging to find out about their side effects and risks. Although economic developments in transatlantic trade fostered the accessibility of coca, prices for the raw product and later cocaine and syringes were too high to be affordable for the wider masses at the beginning. When prices dropped and more people could experience the effects of coca and cocaine on their bodies, more and more articles on the drugs were published through which public opinion could form. Consequently, the sociocultural stage of coca can be situated after that of economy, medicine, and pharmacy but it did not yet call for political action in Britain.

In contrast to other drugs such as opium that had been used in Europe for centuries, access to the novelty drug was limited to the upper classes and the most up-to-date physicians who showed interest in medicinal developments on the continent. Unlike for opium, there existed no broad consumer base until World War I since coca products and later cocaine were still too expensive for the lower classes which fortunately for them, prevented the spread of addiction. Hardly anyone of the working class experienced the effects of those two drugs to foster word-of-mouth recommendation, so the increase in sales resulted primarily from the upper middle and upper classes who were lured by clever advertising of Mariani and others. In fact, coca and later cocaine were the first narcotics that were so extensively advertised, but they experienced comparatively early criticism by the medical profession when dangers became known.

Although the coca and cocaine culture in Britain in the Victorian Era was barely comparable to the opium culture, it is still remarkable how it differed to the coca culture that had existed in South America for millennia. Initially, coca as a novelty on the British market facilitated a 'taste of the exotic' for the upper classes and fostered cultural dissimilation, as examined further down. Reason for that was a changed mode of consumption and the new use as a recreational drug, which also had to do with accessibility. In the eyes of the British, the native coca culture was not civilised enough wherefore they sought to adapt it to their own needs. Part of that was to use coca tonic first and later pure cocaine as a 'mood elevator' that diverged from the drug as merely a medicine to it becoming a luxury indulgence for the rich. Consequently, this also blurred the line between medicinal and recreational use.

The concept of dissimilation in general has primarily been discussed by sociologists and historians of sociology such as Alexander Pinwinkler. According to him, it was crucial that "[...] die negative Abgrenzung vom 'Fremden' eine wesentliche Voraussetzung begründete, um das positive Gegenbild der Angleichung an das 'Eigene' entwerfen zu können. [...] Die ihm von vornherein diskursiv eingeschriebene Kehrseite war die 'Dissimilation' (='Ungleichmachung') des 'Fremden'."[1] It poses a contrast to what ethnologists term assimilation, acculturation, or enculturation in which process people connect with a specific culture, absorb it, and eventually also shape it.[2] Assimilation and dissimilation are not only visible in the way people behave towards other people, they are also visible in the way they embrace or reject each other's cultures and practices. Better tailored to the title of this book, the terms therefore require a specification, wherefore I prefer to speak of cultural dissimilation in the following.

Cultural dissimilation was the most important reason for Britain's unimpressed attitude towards coca and cocaine which it experienced unlike any other narcotic before. This ongoing process describes the rejection of practices and traditions of an inferior culture from a dominant culture. It might result in a preservation of each culture's unique identity but also prevents a

1 Alexander Pinwinkler, "'Assimilation' und 'Dissimilation' in der 'Bevölkerungsgeschichte', ca. 1918 bis 1960," in: *Bevölkerungsforschung und Politik in Deutschland im 20. Jahrhundert*, ed. Rainer Mackensen (Wiesbaden: VS Verlag für Sozialwissenschaften, 2006), 23, 24, transl.: "the negative distinction of the 'otherness' is a crucial requirement to create the positive counter-image of the assimilation to the 'own.' [...] The previously inherent discursive flipside was the 'dissimilation' of the 'otherness.'"

2 Michael Maurer, *Kulturgeschichte* (Köln: Böhlau-Verlag, 2020), 14.

better understanding of the succumbing culture. Various factors such as the level of exposure and social dynamics influence the extent to which cultural dissimilation occurs and if it is a temporal or final event that shapes the non-adopting culture. With Britain being located an ocean away and limiting their relations with South American countries to overseas trade, exposure to coca culture in Peru, for example, was almost non-existent. This fostered cultural dissimilation. In addition, the fact that coca chewing was considered a native and somewhat barbaric habit influenced British society to that extent that it was rejected and had Britons develop their own mode of consumption.[3] Moreover, they used it for other ailments than the natives and it newly discovered alkaloid opened new ways to therapeutic applications which revolutionised surgeries.

Although coca was a cultural marker just like opium in the decades prior, the British sought to distance themselves from associations with populations whose consumption habits they deemed 'barbaric.'[4] Therefore, Britons changed not only their modes of consumption but also their applications as far as possible to prevent association with the indigenous population and their vices. The Inca, for example, originally burnt coca leaves in religious rituals to facilitate communication with the Gods and when coca was allowed for the common people, the habit of coca chewing spread quickly. Just like the conquistadores, the British felt repelled by the native coca chewing, viewing it as not becoming of a civilised Victorian to engage in such a public display of chewing. In addition, the avid British tea drinker also dispensed with drinking coca tea due to the availability of better and more tasteful alternatives.[5] Sim-

---

3 Interestingly, chewing tobacco did not face the same prejudice and remained popular until the expansion of the cigarette industry in the early twentieth century, see IARC Working Group on the Evaluation of Carcinogenic Risks to Humans, "Smokeless Tobacco and Some Tobacco-specific N-Nitrosamines," *IARC Monographs on the Evaluation of Carcinogenic Risks to Humans* No. 89 (2007), accessed 18th June 2025, https://www.ncbi.nlm.nih.gov/books/NBK326503/.

4 Similarly, German scientist Gaedcke noted, coca chewing was "als seine nur dem gemeinen Indianer eigene Gewohnheit[,] verachtet," transl.: "disparaged as a habit pertinent only to the rough Indian." See Gaedcke, *Ueber das Erythroxylin*, 8.

5 Coca tea resembles the flavour of weak peppermint tea. It might therefore not have evoked the same effect as a strong black tea with a high caffeine content, true to the motto: If I cannot taste anything, it cannot have any effect on me.

ilar to opium, coca leaves dissolved in alcohol, preferably in Bordeaux wine, proved the solution: Coca wine drinking was British, coca chewing was not.[6]

This cultural dissimilation also became visible in changed applications of coca. In this aspect, the drug shared some similarities with the most prominent drug of the nineteenth century – opium – which makes for a good comparison to also highlight their differences. Both opium and coca were not used in religious rituals anymore, at least not to the same extent as in their countries of origin, and their consumption was not limited to priests. Opium's sleep-inducing and hallucinogenic properties were still known but its use as a pain-relieving panacea became predominant in the Victorian Era. Similarly, coca became known as a tonic for singers with throat ailments, people with digestive disorders, and people in need of a stimulant although it was initially consumed to sustain hunger and labour and alleviate altitude sickness. It seemed as if the applications of opium became more numerous whereas for coca it became more specific, especially after the introduction of cocaine in medicine.

Whereas opium was widely available and affordable for even the poorest, coca was confined to the well-to-do. This resembled the history of coca in Peru where it was originally confined to priests and the upper classes of the Inca before it became available for everyone. However, the spread of coca to all other classes in Victorian Britain could not occur due to a few restrictions. Even in the late Victorian Era, the supply of coca leaves in Britain was still limited which led to comparatively high prices that the lower classes could not afford, especially not on a regular basis. Comparatively early restrictions on both coca and cocaine – roughly fifty years after their introduction into the British market – as well as an increased awareness for addiction successively prevented them to access these narcotics when prices dropped in the early twentieth century.

In rejecting its original mode of consumption and keeping lower classes from being able to afford it, not only the British but Europeans in general managed to dissimilate coca consumption as much as possible from the traditional coca culture in South America. This cultural dissimilation was intentional to mark the distinction between civilised, moralised, and educated Europeans and the barbaric indigenous population.[7] A changed mode of consumption

6 This argument was similarly posed in Gootenberg, *Andean Cocaine*, 19, 25, 26.

7 As anthropologist Richard Price argued about encounters between the British and indigenous populations: "The dynamic element of two groups reacting to and trying to understand each other [was] missing," "One Big Thing: Britain, Its Empire, and Their Imperial Culture," *Journal of British Studies*, Vol. 45, No. 3 (July 2006), 612.

and application should illustrate that they were more advanced in science and medicine to facilitate such a transformation. But this transformation was also forced by changed geographical and social circumstances: Coca was not needed to alleviate altitude sickness in Britain, neither was it needed to sustain physical labour for those who could afford it. Coca was made to fit into British culture rather than vice versa as it was the case with South American countries where the plant originated.

It becomes clear then that coca also experienced a re-commodification in the late-nineteenth century after the commencement of its transatlantic trade. In the Middle Ages, coca kept its role as a cultural marker solely for the indigenous population while economic interests were limited to local businesses. The first commodification then happened in the sixteenth century when the conquistadores used the plant as a monetary means to pay the native mine workers after which some of them explored the lucrative business of coca trading in South America. Some 300 years later, when Europeans re-discovered coca as a valuable drug and established a continuously increasing overseas trade after the 1860s, coca also became re-commodified. Within only a few years, there were tonics, wines, elixirs, pastilles, and tablets with coca that served a variety of purposes to satisfy patients' needs and illustrated mechanisms of market consumerism. As Price claimed, "[n]ew methods of product advertising, for example, emerged at this moment to foster an imperial patriotism" which included products manufactured in Britain from a novel narcotic.[8] Continuous high prices despite falling procurement costs ensured that those products remained profitable for the pharmaceutical industry.

This commodification was clearly visible in specific coca products whose exotic imagery in advertising evoked a strong response in consumers to have a taste of foreign culture. Marianna Torgovnick called this "the West's fascination with the primitive."[9] One of the most famous examples here is Hall's Coca Wine whose advertisements were strongly reminiscent of colonial attitudes. In one advert, you could see a tropical scenery with palm trees and a waterfall where European soldiers in armour encountered barely dressed Indians. The company even explained this scenery on the bottom as a scene of a book called *Westward Ho* by Charles Kingsley in which "Englishmen [were] crossing the Cordillera" but what a fictional British privateer who arrived at

---

8 Price, "One Big Thing," 616.

9 Marianna Torgovnick, *Gone Primitive: Savage Intellects, Modern Lives* (Chicago: Chicago University Press, 1990), 157.

the Caribbean coast of Venezuela had to do with coca consumption in Peru and Bolivia is questionable.[10] Even more questionable was the other famous advertisement for Hall's coca wine that showed a woman dressed in a yellow and black dress with extravagant headdress, white skin, and red lips.[11] The two-tone background was red and white and the writing resembled calligraphy. Utilising this kind of writing, those colours, and the woman's appearance, this strongly evoked Chinese and Japanese sentiments. As explained in the botanical chapter, coca was never grown in either of these countries and neither was there a broad consumer base that would have rectified this display. Stephen Smith & Co., who produced Hall's coca wine, used this distorted imagery of coca consumers solely for the boost of the sales of their products. As Maurer argued, this contrast of culture and the primitive was typical for the colonial and imperialistic age.[12]

The only exception to this interpretation that united the fascination of the exotic with views somehow conducive to the narrative of the pharmaceutical industry could be found in Mortimer's *History of Coca* published in 1901. In his book, the author speaks of the Inca as "a race highly advanced in civilization" that "were in no way allied to the red men of the North," the "nomadic savages."[13] Mortimer also elevated coca as "'The Divine Plant' of the Incas," as can be read in the title, and described its physiological benefits in no less than five out of sixteen chapters. For this extensive examination he had contacted thousands of men in the medical profession about their knowledge about coca and despite some giving an account useful to his research, the majority "wrote in a frank way, that they knew absolutely nothing of coca."[14] Although Mortimer sought to set the record of coca straight after Poeppig's disparaging view in the early nineteenth century, it is questionable what influence his book had in Britain as it was first published in the United States and later in France in a translated version. Possibly the British pharmaceutical industry refrained from this narrative as it compromised the interpretation of coca as an exotic plant which proved an effective marketing strategy, as explained above.

10 "Hall's Coca Wine: a marvellous restorative," advert, c 1890–1899, Wellcome Collection, accessed 18th June 2025, https://wellcomecollection.org/works/gecumam8/images?id=dbg6hvaw.

11 "Hall's Coca Wine: the elixir of life," advert, c 1916, Wellcome Collection, accessed 18th June 2025, https://wellcomecollection.org/works/snfnu6yt/images?id=b3zyxvfd.

12 Maurer, *Kulturgeschichte*, 30.

13 Mortimer, *History of Coca*, 28, 29.

14 Ibid., xi.

As a result, the interpretation of the indigenous culture in South America in Britain was narrowed to the consumption of coca which portrayed the natives as barbaric drug addicts. This was on the one hand reinforced by the omission of motifs behind coca consumption in the Andes, i.e., alleviating altitude sickness and suppressing hunger during hard labour, and the omission of the value of coca for the Inca in history on the other hand. Comprehensive reports about coca that included those aspects could still be found in botanical or medicinal journals but they were certainly not conducive for the goals of the pharmaceutical industry. The native population and their culture were instrumentalized to increase coca's popularity in Europe through a fascination with the 'exotic.' It is obvious that even in the pharmaceutical industry, Britain upheld its supremacist attitudes at the cost of indigenous populations which reinforced the cultural dissimilation of coca.

Since cultural dissimilation works in both ways for the culture that is dissimilated and the culture that dissimilates, traditional coca-consuming countries deserve another look, too. It is remarkable that although coca culture was dissimilated by the British in their country, it was not assimilated to the new British customs in the originating countries. Besides a short caesura after the Spanish conquest, South American populations did not succumb to 'cultural imperialism' in regard to coca: They neither abandoned their traditions, nor embraced the British ways of consumption and application.[15] Part of that stemmed from coca being a necessity in the Andean surroundings and lacking an equivalent alternative, but it also showed how deeply rooted coca was in native society that it could resist pressure not only by one but two dominant cultures: Spanish and British.

Talking about the motifs for this indigenous resistance, cultural historian Edward Said argued that "[n]o one can deny the persisting continuities of long traditions, sustained habitations, […] but there seems no reason except fear and prejudice to keep insisting on their separation and distinctiveness […]."[16] Nevertheless, it is highly doubtful that coca kept its role in South American cultures because of "fear and prejudice" which the encounter with the Iberians in the sixteenth century had already demonstrated. Initially, the Iberians oppressed the coca habit which contradicts the above claim that they kept the

15 For an explanation and example of cultural imperialism see Vikram Singh Amarawat, "Cultural Imperialism and Travel Writing: Glimpses of Richard Burton's Travelogue," *Proceedings of the Indian History Congress* 77 (2016), 645, 646.

16 Edward Said, *Culture and Imperialism* (New York: Knopf, 1993), 336.

two cultures distinct out of prejudicial feelings of superiority and the desire to maintain hierarchies. This also eliminates the seemingly inferior South American cultures' fear to refrain from cultural exchange in order not to lose their identity – they had to obey the supremacist power. The Iberian change of mind a few years later also contradicts this theory as the decisive arguments lied not in fear and prejudice but in coca being a requirement for mine workers and the drug becoming a lucrative commodity.[17] The latter argument was also the decisive one for British and other European merchants in the nineteenth century which contributed to the coca culture surviving in countries such as Peru and Bolivia to this day.

A more advantageous explanation for the persisting dissimilation of the South American coca culture was given by sociologist Georg Simmel. He claimed that "[e]s entspricht dem zweckmäßigen Instinkt der Masse, dem Wechsel der Umstände und Anregungen gegenüber ihr Selbst durch substanzielle Festigkeit und Unnachgiebigkeit ihrer Form, statt durch schmiegsame Anpassung und rasch eingestellten Wechsel ihres Verhaltens zu bewahren."[18] For Simmel, instinct rather than fear and prejudice was the motif for a society to keep its cultural traditions and practices. Anthropologist Catherine J Allen echoed this stating that "Andean people have shown remarkable resilience in maintaining their way of life in the face of social, religious, and economic forces beyond their control."[19] This argument for cultural dissimilation is more plausible as coca was a necessary commodity in the Andean environment – a circumstance that is still valid until this day. Whether their instinct also accounted for the mode of consumption to remain the same over centuries and not assimilate to Western practices is still up for debate but it contributed to coca's continuous role as a cultural marker.

Another reason for the cultural dissimilation of coca in South American cultures originated in the fact that they became aware of cultural imperialism sooner or later. It often occurred in subtle ways that only showed its influence over time when traditions were eroded or new consumer products entered the

17 This argument was echoed by Christison in "Observations on the Effects of Cuca," 527.

18 Georg Simmel, *Soziologie*, 603, transl.: "it matches the expedient instinct of the crowd to maintain its Self in the face of changing circumstances and stimuli through substantial firmness and rigidity rather than through pliable accommodation and quickly shifting behaviour."

19 Catherine J Allen, "Coca and Cultural Identity in Andean Communities," in: *Coca and Cocaine. Effects on People and Policy in Latin America*, eds. Deborah Pacini and Christine Franquemont (Peterborough: Transcript Printing Company, 1986), 46.

market. In the case of the Spaniards, this was more obvious as they disparaged and forbade coca for a while before realising its importance for the native population. British cultural imperialism, on the contrary, could have led to British products such as coca wine being imported and sold in South American countries but this never reached the same extent as in Europe by far. However, the resistance to this cultural imperialism was visible through the preservation of traditions with coca and the continued practice of chewing coca or drinking it as tea. This was important as it contributed greatly to the preservation of the South American coca culture, as well as the civilisations' identity and history there for which coca has been an important marker.

The process of cultural dissimilation persisted with the discovery of cocaine in the late-nineteenth century. Not only Britain but Europe and North America exploited coca-producing countries, particularly Peru, for the manufacture of cocaine for the Western markets. Comparatively cheap crude cocaine was shipped overseas to produce cocaine-containing drugs that earned the pharmaceutical industry a considerable amount of money. Yet South American countries did not see any benefits from that, neither financially nor in the form of medicinal knowledge. Some historians such as Boucher have argued that the manufacture and trade of crude cocaine has created a profitable industry in the producing countries but it is hardly imaginable that this was a profitable business for all concerned.[20] The numbers he gave for the late twentieth century, namely that coca farmers "receive[d] less than 1.5% of the value for which cocaine [wa]s sold in the United States," most likely did not look that much different in the nineteenth century, if not worse.[21] Even then, South American coca farmers produced a valuable narcotic for the pharmaceutical industries in the Northwestern Hemisphere from which they benefitted neither financially nor medicinally. On the contrary, it would mark the beginning of an illegal industry after the turn of the century that would accelerate the deterioration of public health and morality in those countries.

The cultural dissimilation evolving around coca also cannot shake off supremacist tendencies. Whereas the Peruvian-Britain axis has made this very clear, looking at the Britain-French-German axis illustrates that even further. With the rise of coca products in France, for example *Vin Mariani*, they also gained popularity in Britain. Notable figures greatly promoted sales with their recommendations which led to an increase in imports to Britain.

20 Boucher, "Cocaine and the Coca Plant," 73.

21 Ibid., 76.

Those coca products did not experience a changed mode of consumption but instead had many copycats chasing Mariani's success. When the anaesthetic properties of the valuable alkaloid were then discovered in Germany, Britain took interest in research on the drug and adopted the use of cocaine of anaesthesia in surgery without making any changes. It is obvious that rather than cultural dissimilation, cultural *assimilation* has taken place here. Showing interest in medicinal developments surrounding cocaine on the continent, adopting medical knowledge, and integrating medicinal techniques thereof has contributed to the shaping of modern surgery and patient care in Britain. This was of course welcomed but it showed that assimilating other European practices in British medicine was self-evident whereas assimilating that of South American countries was not.

Pinwinkler claims that the aim of the concept of dissimilation and assimilation was to theoretically reflect practices of social entanglements, provide statistical and empirical evidence and utilise this knowledge for sociopolitical aims in the context of applied sciences.[22] It can be agreed that social entanglements through empirical evidence become more visible through this concept but whether these also rest on statistical evidence is questionable. In the case of coca, numbers are not the crucial point, it is the way people interacted to first make coca a new European commodity, how the new drug was introduced into the British market, and how consumer reacted to it. There are of course Bills of Entry and consular reports that provide statistical data, as Chapter II has shown, but they do not reveal motifs behind social interactions and reasons for cultural changes, such as the changed mode of consumption and application of coca.

Whether this knowledge was conducive for sociopolitical aims is also up for debate. On the one hand, the pharmaceutical industry utilised the fascination for the exotic, and therefore its dissimilation from European practices, as a marketing strategy for coca. Later on, it greatly promoted the newly discovered cocaine for the same reason, as it was not consumed in South America at that time. On the other hand, both drugs did not become a political issue until the early twentieth century, which I elaborate in the last chapter. Ironically, including these in the debate on narcotics stemmed from cultural dissimilation. The rising concern was not over coca being chewed or drunken as tea as in

22 Pinwinkler, "'Assimilation' und 'Dissimilation' in der 'Bevölkerungsgeschichte', ca. 1918 bis 1960," 43.

South American cultures, it was about its alkaloid cocaine being injected subcutaneously and causing addiction which posed a threat to public health, and especially to morality. Consequently, Pinwinkler is right that cultural dissimilation became relevant for sociopolitical aims in the first years of the twentieth century, but not in a conducive way. In the case of coca and cocaine, it backfired. Whereas coca has remained a valuable medicine in Andean societies, cocaine became major commodity in the illicit global narcotics trade.[23]

2. The Novel Narcotic in Popular Culture

Nineteenth-century newspapers and magazines make for an indispensable tool to trace the career of coca in British society and how it compared to that in other countries, especially in Germany. Of particular interest are the articles leading up to this discovery, those published after cocaine's usefulness in ophthalmology and anaesthesia in general, and the time in between, i.e., from 1860 to 1884. The content editors chose to write about influenced public opinion as literacy among the population increased and coca was no exception to that. Newspapers, gazettes, and magazines circulated everywhere, both in the metropolis and the countryside, and often cost as little as one penny which made them affordable even for the lower classes.[24] Medical news, such

---

23 For more information and the most recent statistics on coca (and opium poppy) cultivation, production, and seizures, also in comparison to other narcotics on the market, see: United Nations Office on Drugs and Crime, *Special Points of Interests*, accessed 18th June 2025, https://www.unodc.org/documents/data-and-analysis/WDR_2024/WDR_2024_SPI.pdf, 6, 7.

24 In "The deleterious dominance of The Times in nineteenth-century historiography," *Journal of Victorian Culture* 18 (4) (2013), 481, Andrew Hobbs claims that "[t]he weekly or bi-weekly provincial paper, not the London daily, was the typical Victorian newspaper. There were never more than 20 London morning papers at any one time until the 1890s, while provincial weeklies and bi-weeklies could be counted in their hundreds [...]." However, the reliability, validity, and accuracy of those provincial weeklies are questionable and raise questions as to the usefulness here wherefore they were neglected. The selection of British print media for this chapter was based on circulation, target audience, and, most importantly, relevance to best depict how coca and cocaine were introduced into British society and dealt with over the decades. On one end of the spectrum was the *Morning Chronicle* which was published daily for an affordable 1p in 1865 and targeted liberals as the authors considered themselves "moderate enlightened dissenters." The *Guardian* was slightly less liberal but enjoyed wider

as those about new drugs on the market or innovative treatments, could thus spread easily among all levels of society and more importantly, pharmaceutical companies could advertise their products and thereby increase sales.

The articles on coca and cocaine that were published in British print media should be contrasted with those in German newspapers to elucidate how reports and reactions to those narcotics differed. Germany occupied an exceptional position because it played a crucial role in the rediscovery of coca by explorers in the early nineteenth century, because it was a German chemist who extracted the alkaloid, and because its marvellous properties as an anaesthetic agent were first presented in Germany. Given that the German pharmaceutical industry would become the leader in cocaine production at the end of the Victorian Era, this comparison is reasonable and highlights different perceptions of the development of the two drugs and of their role in both German and British society.[25]

---

circulation despite its rather high price of 2d in 1855. On the other end of the spectrum was the *Morning Post* which, contrary to the uncanny likeness to the title of the former, served the extremely conservative elite. Its price dropped from 4p in 1860 to 1p in 1900 which fostered its circulation that reached over 75.000 at the turn of the century. Joining the ranks of conservative newspapers was the similarly widely circulated and reputable *Times* that put forward noted journalists and the *Pall Mall Gazette* that was intended for "the Gentleman of England." Whereas those publications focused primarily on *Zeitgeschehen*, particularly in politics, the *Strand Magazine* and the *Penny Illustrated* sought to cover other aspects as well, such as nature and technology. They also included more illustrations and less advertising but they were only published monthly for 6p and weekly for 1d, respectively. This range of titles seeks to reflect the attitudes of the British public as best as possible to include different social classes and political views. Compare "Morning Chronicle," The British Newspaper Archive, accessed 18th June 2025, https://www.britishnewspaperarchive.co.uk/titles/morning-chronicle; Wilfrid Hope Hindle, *The Morning Post, 1772–1937: portrait of a newspaper* (London: Routledge, 1974), 218, 240; Hindle, *The Morning Post*, 176; William Makepeace Thackeray, *The History of Pendennis* (London: Smith, Elder & Co, 1887), 345.

25 Since reports on coca were rare before 1860, no specific newspaper titles have been selected for this time and even the news about Niemann's discovery did not make such a big difference. It was only after 1871 that articles and advertising on coca and cocaine increased significantly from about a handful a year to several dozen that were often cross-published. This differed significantly to the marketing of other narcotics such as opium, as they had permeated the British market for decades and thus already assembled a broad consumer base which made advertising in printed media for it redundant. The selection of German newspapers was based on place of publication, area of distribution, and relevance for the career of coca, both in Germany and Britain.

Until 1859, coca received hardly any attention in British print media. Articles on coca in newspaper were rare and any notions were usually limited to listing coca as the "*Narcotic of the Andes*" next to opium, hemp, and other drugs. Nevertheless, two articles stood out at that time as they dealt with coca in more depth.[26] One was "The Coca Chewers of Peru" published in the *London Saturday Journal* in November 1839 which was a very early report based on Poeppig's *Travels*. Due to the author's reliance on Poeppig, it hardly comes as a surprise that he highlighted coca's seemingly deleterious effects on body and mind, particularly on morality, and called people ignorant for "extolling the Coca as a wonderful plant."[27] Moreover, he assured that "the power of the plant [was] only an excitement which soon [became] dangerous" wherefore he agreed with a Spanish chronicler that the consumption of coca would only "fit for the Indians" with their "depraved taste."[28] The other article, published twenty years later in *Blackwood's Edinburgh Magazine*, sought to provide a more balanced view of coca in acknowledging the plant's agricultural, commercial, and social importance for South American populations and explaining its benefits and risks. He also admitted that "[o]f the chemical history of the coca leaf [they were] almost entirely ignorant" wherefore further chemical experiments are required to determine the possibility to introduce it to the European market.[29] The relativization of the perception of coca from the first to the second article stemmed from newly published reports by South American explorers who invalidated Poeppig's descriptions and it showed that there was a chance for coca to be introduced into the British market as a novel narcotic.

At the same time in German newspapers, notions about traditional coca consumption in Peru and the drug's properties to sustain labour and suppress hunger were squeezed into short paragraphs on miscellaneous news that appeared somewhere on the bottom of the last pages.[30] Occasionally, authors mentioned it as a narcotic substance, for example when reviewing James W Johnston's *Naturwissenschaftliche Volksbücher. VII. Die Chemie des täglichen Lebens*

26 "Opium – Opium-Eaters – The Opium-Trade with China," *The Saturday Magazine* (November 1839), 199; "The Narcotics we indulge in," 622–628.

27 "The Coca Chewers of Peru," 327.

28 Ibid., 326, 327.

29 "The Narcotics we indulge in," 626, 627.

30 "Amerika. (Peru.)," *Karlsruher Zeitung* (4th January 1826), 3; "Miszellen. Briefboten in Peru.," *Bonner Zeitung* (22nd March 1826), 4.

in which coca was listed as one of the "narkotischen Stoffe," or when comparing consumers of stimulating brewed beverages.[31] Articles during that time showed that Germans already knew about coca's narcotic properties and some of its effects on the human body but they had not yet considered the drug's usefulness for Europeans. However, the tone was much more informative, interested, and open-minded than that of British authors who sounded devaluating and doubtful of this newly rediscovered narcotic: "We must not forget, if ever it become general in this country, that it has somewhat of a bad reputation (I fear a deserved one), which may counterbalance its virtues."[32]

The number of reports on coca slowly but steadily increased after the *Novara* brought back coca leaves from South America and enabled the extraction of its valuable alkaloid. The *Bonner Zeitung* was one of the first newspapers that extensively reported about the expedition of the *Novara* from which Dr Scherzer brought "fast einen halben Zentner Cocablätter" of which thirty pounds were handed over to Prof Wöhler and his assistant Albert Niemann in September 1859.[33] Several journalists were convinced that coca was destined for something great: "[A]llein schon jetzt ist große Wahrscheinlichkeit vorhanden, daß die Coca zu wichtigen medicinischen Anwendungen berufen sein, und im Handel wie in der Heilwissenschaft noch eine bedeutende Rolle spielen dürfte."[34] Another one wrote that cocaine "verdient gewiß auch in weiteren Kreisen bekannt zu werden" since "der Gegenstand [scheint] in therapeutischer Hinsicht beachtenswerth."[35] As a conclusion, their introduction into the European market could not be recommended enough.[36] References in the reports also showed

31 "Naturwissenschaftliche Volksbücher. VII. Die Chemie des täglichen Lebens," *Aachener Zeitung* (20th April 1855), 3, transl.: "narcotic agents."; "The Chymistry of Common Life," *The Times* (20th January 1855); "Verschiedenes," *Arnsberger Kreisblatt* (9th February 1856), 3, according to which there were ten million coca consumers in comparison to 100 million coffee drinkers.

32 F, "The Coca Plant of Peru.," *The London Reader* (11th May 1867), 28.

33 "Erfolge der Fahrt der "Novara."," *Bonner Zeitung* (4th May 1860), 2, transl.: "almost half a quintal of coca leaves."

34 Ibid., 2, transl.: "Even now the probability is high that coca is destined for important medicinal applications and will play a significant role in commerce as in medicine."

35 "Vermischtes.," *Bonner Zeitung* (4th November 1860), 7, transl.: "certainly deserves to become known in other circles" since "the drug [seems] remarkable in a therapeutic aspect."; "Endlich legte D. Marquart ein Kästchen mit Cocablättern vor...," *Kölnische Zeitung* (15th October 1861), 5.

36 "Die Reihe der anesthetischen (betäubenden) Mittel...," *Echo der Gegenwart* (30th March 1862), 5.

that the Germans followed up with the history of coca, from the Spaniards discovering the plant in the sixteenth century to various explorers, including Poeppig, Tschudi, Weddel, and Mantagazza.[37] They were also aware that "die chemischen Eigenschaften wie die medicinischen Wirkungen des Cocastrauches [waren] in Europa niemals gründlich untersucht worden" although the drug had a long tradition in its country of origin.[38] That was why their joy was even greater that scientists such as Prof Albers in Bonn, Prof Wöhler in Göttingen, and Dr Marquart in Cologne presented fresh coca leaves to the public and briefed the audience about this new stimulant that supposedly ranged between wine and coffee as a semi-luxury food and seemed closest to opium in its pharmaceutical action.[39] From the moment a significant amount of coca leaves entered Germany and revealed a much more potent substance, many Germans – not only scientists but also journalists – seemed to be sure that coca was to become a valuable alkaloid in both the medicinal and recreational world.

The reaction to the discovery of coca's active principle in Britain looked somewhat different and was most likely the result of the discovery not being made by the British. *The London Review*, for example, reported about "A New Stimulant" in 1861 without even mentioning cocaine but presenting coca leaves as a novelty instead.[40] Similarly, the *Journal of the Society of Arts* mentioned the sale of coca wine and elixir in France, but spoke no word of cocaine.[41] Fifteen years later in 1876, another author argued that they could "well be spared another peril" since they "did not need the introduction or spread of a new narcotic amongst our population."[42] Such notions were less reminiscent of ignorance but seemed more a reaction to the bruised ego of the vast and powerful British Empire that was unable to discover this novel narcotic themselves first. This attitude was also the reason why the coca trials by eminent Prof Christison

37 "Vermischtes.," 7; "Ein neues Opiat.," *Echo der Gegenwart* (18th December 1861), 1.

38 "Vermischtes.," 7, transl.: "the chemical properties as well as medicinal effects of the coca shrub had never been thoroughly analysed in Europe."; "Endlich legte D. Marquart," 5.

39 "Niederrheinische Gesellschaft für Natur- und Heilkunde zu Bonn.," *Kölnische Zeitung* (23rd March 1860), 5; "Erfolge der Fahrt der "Novara."," *Bonner Zeitung*, 2; "Endlich legte D. Marquart," 5.

40 "Scientific Intelligence. A New Stimulant.," *The London Review* (14th September 1861), 329.

41 "Cocoa," *Journal of the Society of Arts* (4th September 1868), 728. The author mistakenly added an O when it should have been 'coca.'

42 "A Costly Stimulus.," *Once a Week* (1st April 1876), 51.

in Edinburgh, as described in a previous chapter, were unimposing and British media continued to report that "there was no objective result [in experiments with coca] to encourage its continued administration" because "[o]f stimulants [they had] enough and to spare."[43]

The reminiscence of British supremacy in their dealing with coca in a medicinal, pharmaceutical, and sociocultural context opposed German curiosity and created a hurdle for coca's success in Britain that could have easily been prevented. The *Saturday Magazine* and the *London Saturday Journal*, for example, explained that "[m]any to indulge in its [coca's, KE] use forsake the rational associations of civilized life" and that "the use of the Coca is purely a depraved taste, and only fit for the Indians as they now are."[44] This was also echoed by another correspondent in the *London Reader*.[45] Even Christison, who could confirm some of its benefits, recommended that "no one should use it medicinally" as too little was known about its effect on the human body.[46] This was contradictory to the perception of coca and cocaine on the continent where the two drugs had already been considered valuable additions to the range of narcotics.

In contrast to Britain, Germany looked to other countries for the research on the new narcotic and the first advertisement for coca pills produced by American physician Dr Sampson in Berlin and Braunschweig was published in 1866.[47] It would take Britain another thirteen years to publish their first advert for a coca beverage in a weekly magazine which enabled Germany to greatly increase the popularity of coca products in their country in the meantime.[48] Until 1879, no less than sixteen German newspapers had published coca adverts at least every two weeks, later daily, among them *Echo der Gegenwart*, *Kölnische Zeitung*, *Rhein- und Ruhrzeitung*, *Sächsiche Dorfzeitung*, and *Schwäbischer Merkur*.[49] News about that novelty narcotic spread rapidly and as a result, coca

---

43 "Coca.," *Chamber's Journal of Popular Literature, Science and Arts* no. 646 (13th May 1876), 318; "The Coca-Leaf," *The Times* (24th March 1876), 7.

44 "Opium," *The Saturday Magazine*, 199; "The Coca Chewers of Peru," 327.

45 See footnote 32.

46 Christison, "Observations on the Effects of Cuca," 531.

47 "Neue americanische Medicamente des Special-Arztes Dr. Sampson aus New York," *Kölnische Zeitung* (5th June 1866), 4.

48 ""Coca Leaf."," *The Academy* (11th October 1879), v; "Wordsworth's Coca Leaf," *The Examiner* (29th November 1879), 1554.

49 "Dr. medic. Samson's Coca-Pillen," *Echo der Gegenwart* (13th March 1867), 3; "Lungenleiden, Schwächezustände," *Kölnische Zeitung* (2nd January 1870), 8, "Prof. Dr. Sampson's

could be obtained in no less than twenty-eight apothecaries and pharmacies in Germany but only in one in Britain by 1879.[50] It does not come as a surprise then that coca became an integral part of the pharmacopoeia in Germany much earlier and faster than in Britain which significantly contributed to the latter becoming the centre for pharmaceutical enterprise of cocaine later on.

The lack of reports and research of coca in Britian as well as the scarcity of coca products could therefore not foster a communicative culture about the new narcotic, much in contrast to Germany. In the 1870s, German newspapers fostered the dissemination of knowledge about the plant, arguing that "die merkwürdige Pflanze die volle Aufmerksamkeit insbesondere von medicinischen Autoritäten auf sich zu ziehen verdient" since it was "dem alten Erdtheil immer noch nicht genügend bekannt."[51] The rediscovery of coca as a marvellous drug and the restauration of its reputation had long been overdue according to another newspaper: "[Dr Sampson scheint] den in Amerika seit Jahrtausenden festbegründeten Ruf der Coca auch in Europa wiederhergestellt zu haben, den sie wie keine andere Pflanze in so reichem Maße verdient."[52] There were also contemplations as to the use of coca in the military where it could provide soldiers with strength during forthcoming battles since contempla-

---

Coca Präparate," *Rhein- und Ruhrzeitung* (2nd December 1873), 4; "Prof. Dr. Sampson's Coca Präparate," *Schwäbischer Merkur* (8th July 1873), 6; "Coca Praeparate," *Bonner Zeitung* (8th November 1875), 4.

50 According to coca adverts in *Rhein- und Ruhrzeitung* (30th September 1875), 4; *Neues Tagblatt und General-Anzeiger für Stuttgart und Württemberg* (8th January 1876), 5; *Kölnische Zeitung* (23rd March 1876), 4; *Kölnische Zeitung* (30th August 1876), 7; and *Echo der Gegenwart* (17th September 1876), 4, coca products could be obtained here: J B Becker, Köln; Sellerbeck, Mülheim a. d. Ruhr; Hirschapotheke, Stuttgart; Marienapotheke, Hannover; Dr Schulze and Gebrüder Gehrig, Berlin; Mauritius-Apotheke and Ferdinand Kästner, Cöln; Lotterer & Speidel and Zahn & Seeger, Stuttgart; Fr. Kober and Engelapotheke, Heilbronn; C F Paulsen, Elberfeld; Dr H Kühlze and M Fickeissen and Dr R Puller, Crefeld; Löwenapotheke, Reutlingen; Mohrenapotheke, Ulm; G Hölzke, Düsseldorf; C Fuchs, Coblenz; Wilhelm Rump, Dortmund; G A Schäffer, Cleve, A Pick, Ahrweiler; R Straßburger, Saarlouis; J P Müller, Hörde.

51 "Ein wunderbares Kräftigungsmittel," *Leipziger Tageblatt und Anzeiger* (3rd October 1874), 9, transl.: "the peculiar plant deserves full attention, particularly from medicinal authorities" since it was "still unknown to the old continent."

52 "Coca-Präparate," *Karlsruher Zeitung* (6th April 1873), 3, transl.: "[Dr Sampson seems] to have restored in Europe the millennial-old firm reputation of coca in America which the plant deserves abundantly."

tions about side effects or dangers were still non-existent.[53] Only once did a reader attempt to criticise the new narcotic by asking "Besitzen die viel angepriesenen 'Coca-Präparate' zum Theil wirklich die angelobten Wunderkräfte, oder ist Alles, wie so vieles Andere, nur Schwindel?" but this question got lost in the letterbox section of a newspaper page without being further discussed or at least publicly answered.[54]

The actual juggernaut for reports on coca, however, was the marvellous discovery of cocaine as a local anaesthetic, which was also the first local anaesthetic in general. Whereas the *Lancet* published a translation of Koller's speech before the Vienna Royal Imperial Society of Physicians about two months after it was given, British print media displayed a very reserved reaction in not focusing on recent developments in medicine.[55] There was only one article in *The Glasgow Herald* that was published shortly after and informed the public about the newly discovered anaesthetic in greater depth and a brief paragraph in the *Manchester Times*. The former felt it was their obligation to spread knowledge about such a precious new drug, that "great boon [that] has thus unquestionably been conferred on suffering humanity," since "[t]he progress of medical science and research is a matter in which the public are bound to take a deep and lasting interest, for the plain reason that such progress affects in the most intimate manner the wellbeing of mankind."[56] In taking on such a position, the author of the *Glasgow Herald* article posed an exception in Britain as the absence of articles on Koller's discovery showed. Even the small paragraph published in the *Manchester Times* refrained from giving Koller full credit, stating that "this anaesthetic was discovered recently by accident," merely listing him in a row with other scientists such as Alfred Vulpian, and arguing that the plant should be named cuca instead of coca because this was what Christison had proposed some year prior.[57] Once again, this confirms that the British were sour over Germany being the beacon in cocaine research.

This is especially obvious when contrasting the British reaction to the news in 1884 with the reaction in German newspapers. The novel anaesthetic co-

---

53 "Das neue Heft der Annales du Commerce extérieur...," *Schwäbischer Merkur* (3rd November 1866), 4; "Eine wunderbare Pflanze," *Dresdner Nachrichten* (15th November 1866), 2.

54 Albert B, "Besitzen die viel angepriesenen...," *Dresdner Nachrichten* (17th May 1875), 1, transl.: "Do the much praised "coca preparations" indeed partly possess the lauded miraculous effects or is everything, as many other things, mere quackery?"

55 Koller, "On the Use of Cocaine for producing Anaesthesia on the Eye."

56 "Cocaine," *The Glasgow Herald* (26th December 1884), 6.

57 "Chlorhydrate of Cocaine as an Anaesthetic," *Manchester Times* (6th December 1884), 9.

caine was covered by half a dozen newspapers that reported about a "stürmische Nachfrage nach Cocain, daß binnen wenigen Wochen Alles, was sich von Cocablättern in Europa [...] vorfand, zu irgend steigenden Preisen aufgekauft und verarbeitet wurde, so daß jetzt auch zum 4–5fachen des früheren Werthes nichts mehr zu beschaffen war."[58] Over the next year, Germany discussed prices of cocaine, considered it as a therapy for seasickness and morphine addiction, and even shed light on experiments to synthetically produce cocaine due to the costly extraction from coca leaves.[59] According to those sources, the price for cocaine ranged between 8 and 129 Mark per one gram but that was expected to decrease with the arrival of higher imports of coca leaves. Germany took a much deeper interest in cocaine and was much more engaged in the potential benefits for mankind than Britain and wanted the public to know.

It took one-and-a-half more years until *Chamber's Journal* stated that "Cocaine flashed like a meteor before the eyes of the medical world, but, unlike a meteor, its impressions have proved to be enduring."[60] Nevertheless, these 'enduring impressions' were already fading as criticism of the new narcotic grew, first in Germany but soon after in Britain as well. Roughly a year after Koller published his ground-breaking research, the *Hannoversche Kurier* warned of a "Cocainomanie" that had apparently spread in North America and that the replacement therapy for morphine addicts had the effect of producing a co-dependency rather than curing the patient.[61] This was also highlighted by another author in the *Berliner Volksblatt* who made a dramatic statement saying that "Beelzebub hat den Teufel ausgetrieben, aus dem Morphinisten ist ein – Cocainist geworden."[62] The situation in America seemed to have sparked increasing concerns over cocaine consumption which was visible in headlines such as

58 "Eine lebhafte Conjunctur war für Cocain...," *Leipziger Tageblatt und Anzeiger* (24th April 1885), 17, transl.: "fierce demand for cocaine that within a few weeks all coca leaves that could be found in Europe were sold to increasing prices and manufactured so that even now nothing could be procured for four- and fivefold of the previous value."

59 *Hannoverscher Kurier* (14th November 1884), 3; *Hannoverscher Kurier* (11th April 1885), 5; *Schwäbischer Merkur* (20th November 1884), 15; *Hallesches Tageblatt* (15th February 1885), 2; "(Ein neues Mittel gegen die Seekrankheit.)," *Hannoverscher Kurier* (18th November 1885), 6; "Cocain," *Hallesches Tageblatt* (19th December 1885), 4; "Die Herstellung des Cocains...," *Hallesches Tageblatt* (29th December 1885), 2.

60 "Cocaine," *Chamber's Journal*, 147.

61 "(Zur Warnung)," *Hannoverscher Kurier* (3rd December 1885), 6.

62 "In der Cocainnarkose," *Berliner Volksblatt* (24th August 1888), 5, transl.: "Casting out devils by Beelzebub, a morphinist has become – a cocainist."

"Der Fluch der Betäubungsmittel" and "Die Sklaven des Cocain" which could have equally made it onto the thriller bestseller list. Reason for that was an article in an American newspaper in which a doctor described cocaine as the biggest threat to mankind: "Man hatte, wie gesagt, allgemein angenommen, daß kein Mittel den Menschen noch tiefer erniedrigen könne [als Opium und Morphium]. Und doch ist ein solches allem Anscheine nach in dem vielgepriesenen Cocain gefunden worden."[63]

Although the American report did not have seemed to have made it into British newspaper or journals, the British medical profession was well aware that "a potency for good implies a potency for harm," and cocaine proved no exception to that.[64] J B Mattison, a physician writing articles for the *Lancet*, stated that "[s]urely it is high time to draw the line, to revoice a warning as to the use and abuse of this valued but at the same time toxic drug."[65] Of particular concern were the observations by Dr Paul Regnard at a lecture at the Sorbonne who reminded the audience of his words five years prior: "Here is another poison [i.e., cocaine, KE]; it is still new, and consequently little used – in other words, it has not yet become the fashion to employ it. But, depend on it, one of these days we shall have to deal with cocainism."[66] Shocked he added that he "glaubte damals nicht, daß [s]eine Prophezeiung so bald in Erfüllung gehen würde. Es [war] aber in der That so."[67]

Despite Dr Regnard's description of the dangers of cocaine consumption, Britain seemed not as worried about it as Germany. Evidence in newspapers show that Britain did not fully grasp the possibility that cocaine consumption could become a habit and endanger society as a whole. Rather than that, articles in British newspapers reported about singular incidents where somebody had accidentally overdosed a prescription or committed suicide with the help of the drug.[68] Sometimes, law cases emerged where patients sued their doctors for improper treatment with cocaine, as in Freeman v. Ebenezer, Farvish

---

63 "Der Fluch der Betäubungsmittel," *Hannoverscher Kurier* (11th July 1886), 6, transl.: "It was generally assumed that no drug could humiliate humanity more [than opium and morphine]. Yet still it appears that it has been found in the much-lauded cocaine."

64 Mattison, "Cocaine Dosage and Cocaine Addiction," 1024.

65 Ibid., 1024, 1026.

66 "The Use of Cocaine," *The Birmingham Daily Post* (27th December 1889), 5.

67 "Der Cocainismus," *Kölnische Zeitung* (18th December 1889), 1, transl.: "did not believe back then that his prophecy would be fulfilled so very soon. Yet it has indeed."

68 "Suicide with Cocaine," *The Daily News* (9th April 1896), 2; "The supposed Death from Cocaine," *The Daily News* (14th October 1896), 6.

v. Seifert, or Taylor and Wife v. The London Hygienic Institute but that did not affect public opinion much.[69] Warning as to the production of "a special form of mania" evolving from "a form of chronic poisoning produced from the taking of small doses of cocaine daily" were limited to medical journals and medical professionals and did not receive the attention they deserved, thus delaying discussion about restrictions on the sale of cocaine until after the turn of the century.[70]

Meanwhile, Germany did not become weary of reporting about the rapid spread of 'Cocainomanie' or 'Cocainismus.' Physicians, such as Dr Hans Otto, warned of "die übermäßige oder vorschriftswidrige Anwendung" that fostered the "weitere Ausbildung der neuen drohenden Seuche" but also emphasised the role of medical professionals who could prevent that from happening.[71] His colleague Dr Émile Magitot from Paris similarly advocated caution when applying cocaine but believed prohibition would be the wrong way for a narcotic so potent in medicine.[72] It seemed as if Germany gave much more credit to its physicians and their warnings than Britain and did not shy away to inform the public that the physicians themselves ran a significant higher risk to succumb to the cocaine habit.[73] As German journalists remarked: "Auch das viel-

---

69 In all three cases, dentists were sued for cocaine poisoning and the death of a plaintiff's wife that resulted from improper administration. After hearing testimony, the court ruled that all three dentists were not guilty of these allegations. See "Oxford Circuit," *The Times* (11th July 1904), 3; "High Court of Justice. King's Bench Division. The Sale of an Asthma Remedy," *The Times* (16th January 1908); "The Sale of an Asthma Remedy," *The Times* (18th January 1908), 3; "Inquest. Cocaine for Tooth Extraction," *The Times* (23rd January 1908), 5; "The Use of Cocaine," *The Times* (4th September 1908), 2; "King's Bench Division. Taylor and Wife v. The London Hygienic Institute. Alleged Negligent Administration of an Anaesthetic," *The Times* (3rd November 1908).

70 Alexander Blyth, *Poisons: Their Effects and Detection. A Manual for the Use of Analytical Chemists and Experts* (London: Charles Griffin and Company 1895), 349.

71 "Kunst, Wissenschaft und Leben," *Kölnische Zeitung* (13th September 1889), 1, transl.: "the excessive or improper application" that fostered the "further spread of the new threatening epidemic."; Hans Otto, "Warnung vor dem Cocain," *Hagener Zeitung* (9th September 1890), 3; "Cocainismus," *Dresdner Nachrichten* (27th February 1889), 11; "Die Gefährlichkeit mancher modernen Heilmittel," *Berliner Börsen-Zeitung* (20th August 1889), 5.

72 "Arzneikunde," *Dresdner Journal* (15th May 1891), 3.

73 "Ueber die traurigen Folgen der Cocainomanie," *Emscher Zeitung* (3rd November 1888), 5; "Erkenntnisse eines Cocainisten," *General-Anzeiger für Dortmund und die Provinz Westfalen* (19th December 1896), 5.

gerühmte Cocain stellt sich nun, wie uns mitgetheilt wird, leider als ein Danaergeschenk für die Heilwissenschaft heraus. Von verschiedenen Seiten wird bereits über Vergiftungen berichtet [...]. Noch weit schlimmer ist indessen, daß in Amerika bereits eine der Morphiumkrankheit ähnliche, aber noch schrecklichere "Cocainomanie" aufgetaucht ist."[74] Besides of North America, Germany also turned to other countries to support their claim of the spread of a cocaine habit:

> Aus Indien kommt jetzt die Nachricht, daß die Cocainsucht unter den dortigen Einwohnern einen besorgniserregenden Umfang angenommen hat, so daß Maßnahmen zu ihrer Bekämpfung dringend verlangt werden. [...] Auch unter den Negern der Vereinigten Staaten hat übrigens die Cocainsucht eine gefährliche Ausdehnung angenommen, befördert durch die oft ganz übertriebenen Ansprüche, die an die Arbeitsleistung der Neger gestellt werden [...].[75]

In the dawn of the Opium Commission convening in early 1908, a German newspaper thus concluded: "Cocaine! Lautlos, unaufhaltsam, stetig wachsend, hat sich der Gebrauch von Cocain in seiner unheilvoll giftigen Wirkung in Leben und Schicksal Tausender von Menschen eingedrängt, nicht nur in England, sondern auch in Indien und besonders bei den Amerikanern."[76]

Although the expansion of the press and increasing literacy made newspapers more accessible to the general public and therefore contributed to debates about coca entering the public sphere, medical journals played an important role as well. The two most prominent titles that emerged in the Victorian Era

74 "(Zur Warnung)," *Hannoverscher Kurier* (3rd December 1885), 6, transl.: "Even the much-praised cocaine, as we are informed, now turns out to be a Greek gift for medicine. Many sources already report about posionings [...]. Still worse is that an illness resembling morphinism, called cocainomania, has now appeared in America."

75 "Das mörderische Cocain," *Bielefelder General-Anzeiger* (16th January 1903), 6, transl.: "From India we receive news that the addiction to cocaine among the inhabitants has reached a concerning extent so that controlling measures are urgently demanded. [...] The addiction to cocaine has also reached a dangerous extent among the negroes of the United Stated which was fostered by oftentimes very exaggerated demands of the work of the Negroes."

76 "Im Bannes des Cocain," *General-Anzeiger der Stadt Mannheim und Umgebung* (31st January 1908), 11, transl.: "Cocaine! Silently, unstoppable, steadily increasing has the habit of cocaine in its inauspicious poisonous effects intruded the fate and lives of thousands of people, not only in Britain, but also in India, and especially in America."

were the *Lancet* and the *British Medical Journal* (BMJ). Reports on coca in both journals were scarce and only occurred after 1876 when Christison's report on coca was published in the *BMJ*.[77] Koller's discovery of cocaine as an anaesthetic in 1884 then had a much higher impact when in successive years until 1912, the *Lancet* published over 100 articles on the drug itself, as compared to merely over a dozen in the *BMJ*.[78] Nevertheless, both journals mentioned the two drugs in passing in roughly 2000 research articles, news, or correspondence which illustrated that their application in medicine and science had been discussed regularly. Still, the intended audience and content of the articles varied which was reflected in the amount and kind of articles on coca and cocaine they published over the years.

The *BMJ* was initially intended to serve provincial practitioners, as its original title *Provincial Medical and Surgical Journal* highlighted.[79] Even as it expanded its audience, it remained a source for physicians and surgeons primarily seeking practical advice in the form of case studies, clinical guidance, and news about medical advancements or scientific research. This emphasis on practice rather than theory and its measured tone aimed at improving medical science and practice as a whole which greatly differed from the *Lancet*'s goals. The *Lancet* was established as a journal to advocate medical reforms both within the medical profession and society.[80] Its target group was therefore not only physicians and surgeons, but also people outside of the medical field who were interested in medical issues. As a result, publications in the *Lancet* were more confrontational in tone, for example when covering medical malpractice, which sparked debates and could foster reforms.

These differences became evident when coca and cocaine were mentioned in both journals' publications. In the *BMJ*, hundreds of articles between 1884 and 1912 dealt with cocaine being used as an anaesthetic in surgeries, particularly in ophthalmology, laryngology, pharyngology, gynaecology, and obstetrics. Physicians and surgeons described what kind of solution they used, how

77 Christison, "Observations on the Effects of Cuca."

78 See the *BMJ* archive, https://www.bmj.com/archive, and the *Lancet*'s archive, accessed 18th June 2025, https://www.thelancet.com/search/advanced?SeriesKey=lancet&ISSN=0140-6736&journalCode=lancet, when searching for key terms "coca" or "cocaine" in titles.

79 "History of the BMJ," The BMJ, accessed 18th June 2025, https://www.bmj.com/about-bmj/history-of-the-bmj.

80 "About *The Lancet*," The Lancet, accessed 18th June 2025, https://www.thelancet.com/lancet/about.

they applied it, and what effect it had, thus providing colleagues with practical advice about the use of the drug in specific cases.[81] A thorough debate about cocaine's benefits or risks was absent in these articles and negative connotations such as the danger of addiction only occurred after 1900 in a few instances.[82] This stood in sharp contrast to publications in the *Lancet* which already warned against cocaine in the 1880s, almost at the same time it was discovered.[83] In this journal, cocaine was not treated as a means to an end but as a narcotic itself that it was. Consequently, this led to more well-informed readers and wider influence on public opinion than that of the *BMJ*'s.

Newspapers were the first to pick up on coca as a novel narcotic and they were also the ones who informed the public about the discovery of its more potent alkaloid cocaine. Rather than debates surrounding the two drugs making it out there from the medical field, other factors contributed to this development. These were first and foremost the previously examined advertising campaigns which often featured prominent figures and therefore caught more public attention than articles in medical journals – even though the *Lancet* addressed a broader audience.[84] Later on, reports on legal cases, such as malpractice involving cocaine, additionally contributed to bringing the medical debate surrounding the drug into public discourse.[85] Societal movements, such as the temperance movements which I discuss further down, similarly contributed to that in adding coca and cocaine to their list of forbidden intoxicants. The anticipation that the debate surrounding coca and cocaine's potential health risks entered the public sphere from the medical field was therefore only partly applicable, as it was the press, legal cases, and societal circumstances that brought the issue to wider attention.

The years in between the meeting of the commission in Shanghai 1908 and the International Opium Convention 1912 were then characterised by a scarcity of articles on the topic in British print media. A short paragraph squeezed onto

81 See, for example, "Cocaine as a Local Anaesthetic." *British Medical Journal* (6th December 1884): 1161–1162; Alexander Jamieson, "Thomas's Operation for Removal of Benign Tumour of the Female Breast," *British Medical Journal* (9th June 1888): 1216–1217.

82 See, for example, Bose, "Cocaine Intoxication and its Demoralizing Effects."

83 Taylor, "The Dangers of Cocaine," 1070.

84 See footnote 80. The first adverts for coca products in British newspapers appeared in 1879, during a time when neither the *BMJ* nor the *Lancet* published reports specifically on coca or cocaine.

85 See footnote 69 for legal cases.

the last page of *The Times* explained that "[t]he British government [...] yesterday accepted in principle the American invitation to participate in a conference at The Hague in 1911 to consider the regulation of the traffic in opium, cocaine, and morphine" and despite its informative nature appeared to be of no greater importance.[86] It is possible that at least for some British people the conference did not receive as much attention since they regarded their hegemony in the global drug trade as unimpeachable. This arrogance was also visible in their demand that the participating governments should "investigate the manufacture and trade in those things so as to be in a position to deal effectively in the matter" which implied their demand that other countries had to do their homework on drugs first to effectively contribute to the conference.[87]

he concerns evolving around cocaine and other narcotics as a threat to public health received little attention from the British until the first years of the twentieth century and stood in sharp contrast to their covering of the International Opium Convention. Between December 1911 and January 1912, a *Times* correspondent regularly reported about the scope, programme, objects, process, and difficulties of the proceedings to keep the public up to date.[88] This did not come as a surprise as the conference posed a landmark event in the history of narcotics and the questions discussed affected several nations across the globe for decades to come. Nevertheless, if Britain would have covered the conference to that extent if it had not been involved and affected by the decisions made in early 1912 remains questionable.

The situation for Britain at the dusk of the Victorian Era thus looked somewhat different than that of Germany and was certainly incomparable to that in the United States. Whereas most of the countries participating in the convention were worried about the spread of a cocaine habit in their home countries, Britain was more worried about the spread in their colonies than in their motherland. As the previous delineation of the spread of coca and cocaine consumption has shown, there did not seem to be reason for concern. In contrast to the US, Britain did not have to deal with an influx of Chinese immigrants that

86 "Great Britain and the Opium Traffic," *The Times* (22nd September 1910), 5.

87 "Great Britain and the Opium Traffic," *The Times* (22nd September 1910), 5.

88 "The Opium Conference. Meeting at the Hague," *The Times* (2nd December 1911), 5; "The Opium Conference. Its Objects and Programme," *The Times* (11th December 1911), 5; "The Opium Conference. Conclusion of an Agreement," *The Times* (6th January 1912), 6; "The Opium Conference. Causes of Delay," *The Times* (16th January 1912), 5; "The Opium Convention," *The Times* (14th February 1912), 9.

continued their narcotic habits in their new home, or with thousands of black workers that sought refuge in cocaine to endure hard labour. There were some incidents in which cocaine was wrongly applied – whether purposefully, negligently, or ignorantly – or when someone used it to terminate their own life but it did not appear as an unstoppable habit as in other countries. Even in India and Ceylon, where a cocaine habit was said to be on the rise, this merely added to the prevalent opium habit that had already undergone several restrictions by the Indian government in previous decades. Given these circumstances, it is not surprising that there existed a significant lack of data regarding the circulation of cocaine in both Britain and its colonies and that a *Cocaine Committee* to investigate the matter was only established *after* the Opium Convention in 1908.

To Britain's defence, though, a few circumstances contributed to that apparent carelessness. As pointed out in the beginning of this chapter, interest in research of coca and cocaine in Britain started relatively late and did not by far reach the extent as it did in Germany. Whether they decided to leave the field to Germany or were plainly not interested in the rediscovered drug is still up for debate. The answer might lie somewhere in between: The British were indeed interested in coca, as the botanical and economic chapters have shown, but they also realised that they could not compete with Germany who always was a step ahead in terms of trade and pharmaceutical development, as described in this and the previous chapter. However, it is a fact that these circumstances caused a lag in knowledge about the novel narcotic that entailed both positive and negative consequences. On the one hand, the introduction of coca and cocaine products into British society occurred much later than in France, for example, which delayed them becoming popular remedies sooner. The high price also made them primarily a medicinal product whose regular use was confined to those who could afford it. As a result, a potential cocaine habit could not spread as easily as, let's say, an opium habit. On the other hand, delaying the dissemination of knowledge about this new narcotic also meant a delay in public awareness of the dangers and risks. As time went by, this became a big problem for those few who light-heartedly indulged in cocaine as a recreational drug.

3. Coca(ine) in the World of Fiction

Coca culture also did not skip literature, especially after cocaine became known as a stimulant for the brain. In fiction, authors often incorporated drug use in their works to shed light on the destructive nature of narcotics that formed the darker side of society and humanity in general, as I explain further down. In doing so, they increased public awareness of the dangers of those drugs and fostered awareness about addiction, which was still a relatively new concept at the time. Whereas the portrayal of figures was often exaggerated, they still visualised that even sophisticated and bright individuals were not immune to the negative consequences of narcotic consumption. On the contrary, pursuing pleasure without restraint with the help of drugs could lead to self-destructive and criminal behaviour.

A new genre emerging in the Victorian Era that often borrowed from narcotic cultures to set the tone and create a mystical atmosphere was detective fiction. One of the most prominent examples here is Sir Arthur Conan Doyle whose stories revolving about a genius detective called Sherlock Holmes contained several references and explicit passages about narcotic consumption by the main character that were inspired by the author's experience as a physician. Other authors of fiction who included direct or indirect references to narcotic consumption were Robert Louis Stevenson and Oscar Wilde who contributed to an increased awareness for the risks and dangers of narcotics in society and thus influenced public opinion.

From those authors, Conan Doyle stood out as he had a medicinal background that influenced his writings. In the late 1870s, he studied medicine at the University of Edinburgh to become a physician and during his five years in Scotland, he must have made acquaintance of Sir Robert Christison, a professor of medicine at the university, and heard of his experiments with coca. After opening and closing unsuccessful practices in Plymouth and Portsmouth, in between which he continued writing, Conan Doyle took increased interest in ophthalmology. It is highly likely that the discovery of cocaine as the first local anaesthetic in 1884 sparked his curiosity which culminated in a visit to Vienna in 1891 to expand his knowledge. Ensuing from Christison's trials, Conan Doyle must have kept track of coca's career in successive years and was probably fascinated by its evolution as a medical marvel. Although he did not stay in Vienna for long, he must also have come across Sigmund Freud, who lectured at the University in Vienna and had published “Ueber Coca” a few years prior.[89]

After 1887, Doyle became most famous with the four novels and fifty-six short stories he wrote about detective Sherlock Holmes whom he portrayed as an ingenious mastermind and drug addict. He craftily interwove his medicinal knowledge and experience he gained in Edinburgh and Vienna into his stories which made them more realistic than other works in the genre. This medicinal background became most visible in “The Man with the Twisted Lip” when Doyle called Thomas De Quincey, author of *Confessions of an English Opium-Eater*, a “foolish freak” and “wreck and ruin of a noble man.”[90] Later in the story, Dr Watson encountered his companion Sherlock Holmes in an opium den where Holmes wondered if Watson “imagine[d] that [he had] added opium-smoking to cocaine injections.” Watson himself explained that he was “holding [his] breath to keep out the vile, stupefying fumes of the drug [i.e., opium].”[91] In *The Sign of Four*, Doyle’s medicinal knowledge became most visible:

> Sherlock Holmes took his bottle from the corner of the mantlepiece, and his hypodermic syringe from its neat morocco case. With his long, white, nervous fingers he adjusted the delicate needle and rolled back his left shirt-cuff. […] Finally, he thrust the sharp point home, pressed down the tiny piston, and sank back into the velvet-lined armchair with a long sigh of satisfaction. […] “Which is it to-day?” I asked, “morphine or cocaine?” […] “It is cocaine,” he said, “a seven-per-cent-solution. […]”[92]

Such notions could not have come from an average writer since many had never made it to an opium den or witnessed addiction to both opium and cocaine. They mostly relied on few reports in newspapers and magazines which often led to exaggerations or distortions, for example, that the East End in London was crowded by opium dens operated by the Chinese.

Doyle’s words, however, showed that he had detailed knowledge about the kind of narcotics that were consumed, how they were consumed, and what effects they had on the human body. As opium was omni-present, this it hardly surprising, but opium-smoking was not as common and neither was cocaine

---

89 Freud,“Ueber Coca;” Jakob Lehne, “Arthur Conan Doyle in Wien,” Wien Museum, accessed 18th June 2025, https://magazin.wienmuseum.at/arthur-conan-doyle-in-wien.

90 Doyle, “The Man with the Twisted Lip,” 623.

91 Ibid., 626–7.

92 Doyle, *The Sign of Four*, 1–3.

consumption. His vivid description of an opium den and detailed description about narcotic consumption points towards him knowing about this from personal experience, but his disparaging choice of words in "Twisted Lip," as mentioned above, indicate that this was more 'observing' rather than 'consuming' experience. Doyle as a physician would have certainly witnessed the effects of narcotics on his patients, but due to his ill success in this profession, it is questionable whether he ever possessed cocaine injections or applied them in his practice. D N Pearce argued that part of that knowledge stemmed from conferences of the British Dental Association in Doyle's hometown who regularly discussed cocaine's role in dentistry.[93] It is safe to say, though, that he knew about the mind-expanding and exhilarating effects of cocaine injections that were crucial for his portrayal of Sherlock Holmes as an investigative genius.

In doing so, Doyle combined two paradoxes that initially were not thought to go together: narcotics and ingenuity. For decades, if not centuries, opium consumption was associated with the working class as it became a daily necessity for most of them and contributed to moral and physical deterioration. Opium did not foster morality but destroyed it, so it was as far from ingenuity as can be. Similarly, cocaine was first and foremost a local anaesthetic and not a luxury stimulant for the brain. If anything, it was considered a stimulant for the body but not a drug to increase one's intellectual capabilities. Through Sherlock Holmes, Doyle suggested that narcotics can have positive effects on the mind but that they were accompanied by side effects, nonetheless. Explained his famous creation:

> My mind[, he said,] rebels at stagnation. Give me problems, give me work, give me the most abstruse cryptogram or the most intricate analysis, and I am in my own proper atmosphere. I can dispense then with artificial stimulants. But I abhor the dull routine of existence. I crave for mental exaltation. That is why I have chosen my own particular profession, or rather created it, for I am the only one in the world.[94]

This quote clearly showed that Doyle saw a connection between "artificial stimulants" and "mental exaltation" and that he believed some stimulants could help escape "the dull routine of existence." In putting these words in Holmes' mouth,

93 D N Pearce, "Sherlock Holmes, Conan Doyle and Cocaine," *Journal of the History of Neuroscience* (1994), 227.

94 Doyle, *The Sign of Four*, 4, 5.

the author was most likely inspired by Freud who was the first to speak highly and publicly of the great benefits of recreational cocaine use and, to a lesser extent, of his fascination for spiritualism.

Throughout his stories, Doyle did not use the word addiction, but he was aware of the habit-forming nature of narcotics that was the forerunner of the concept of addiction. As he noted in *The Sign of Four*, Holmes' forearm and wrist were "all dotted and scarred with innumerable puncture-marks" and Watson mentioned witnessing the performance of cocaine injections "[t]hree times a day for many months."[95] What was initially a vice, became known as a habit but it took medicine a few decades to develop an actual concept of addiction that constituted an illness that had to be treated.[96] Doyle contributed to this development since he portrayed his detective not only as a brilliant thinker but also an addict whose health deteriorated with his drug consumption. In telling the stories from Dr Watson's perspective, Doyle could not disguise autobiographical influences, and he let his character speak freely about what he thought of narcotics such as opium, morphine, and cocaine.

Doyle's works on Sherlock Holmes also reflected the medicinal progress in the last years of the nineteenth century that shed light on the dangerous sides of narcotic consumption. He was not the only author who did so. A fellow writer from Scotland, Robert Louis Stevenson, also processed narcotic consumption in one of his most famous works published in 1886: *Strange Case of Dr Jekyll and Mr Hyde*. The story about the respectable and good-hearted physician Dr Jekyll who turns into choleric and terrifying Mr Hyde at night dealt with a variety of themes, one of which was addiction. Whereas Stevenson never explained what drug Dr Jekyll took that initiated his transformation, the effects it had can be associated with opiates and cocaine, although the mysterious drug could also have been a hallucinogenic mushroom. Leaving the question for the kind of drug aside, the author wanted to raise the reader's awareness for the risks of narcotics if taken in excess. In a similar way, this is also visible in Dorian Gray, Oscar Wilde's vain and youth-obsessed character who dies after stabbing his aging self-portrait. While addiction was not a main theme in Wilde's novella, Gray's visits to an opium den due to his "hideous hunger for opium [beginning] to gnaw at him" and his hedonistic, amoral, and narcissistic personality implied that those with an over-indulgence in opium become obnoxious mem-

95 Ibid., 2.

96 More on the evolution of the concept of addiction further down.

bers of society.[97] All three authors can be considered examples of a new thinking of narcotic consumption that was a one-eighty turn from De Quincey's *Confessions* from 1821 and reflected a development in society as a whole.

Sherlock Holmes, Mr Hyde, and Dorian Gray were not the stereotypical addicts in the Victorian Era because they were members of at least the upper middle class. Their explicitly ascribed addiction helped authors to draw a connection between narcotics and morality which obviously, should demonstrate that the former is bad influence for the latter. What is remarkable, though, is that the social background of these characters differed from the ones that were usually considered addicts. No longer were it the Chinese Lascars or the working-class mothers who sedated their babies for a long day at work, but they were respectable, well-known members of society who fell victim to their cravings. The resulting deterioration of morality showed that this no longer effected only the poor and uneducated but that it became a problem for the middle and upper classes as well, and one that was voiced.

All three, Doyle, Stevenson, and Wilde, increased the public's consciousness for addiction since they were the most popular British authors who critically processed narcotic consumption in their works. Out of the three, Doyle was the only one through which cocaine gained centre stage and it was thanks to his medical background that his descriptions were the most accurate and reliable. This was important as many contemporary sources were biased towards narcotics which led to exaggerations or downplaying their effects. Whereas this was certainly not enough to speak of the creation of a so-called coca or cocaine culture in Britain, his works illustrated that cocaine was not an unknown narcotic purified from an exotic South American plant anymore. Doyle demonstrated that the understanding of coca and cocaine slowly but surely progressed from medicinal to recreational drug in modern terms. This was also true for opium in the other authors' works where the motif for narcotic intake lay outside a medicinal necessity. Whereas some scholars doubt that Doyle had such a significant influence on cocaine awareness, one should not underestimate his contribution – especially since for many the stories about Sherlock Holmes were the first detailed accounts of cocaine administration and -addiction they heard of or read about.

97 Oscar Wilde, *The Picture of Dorian Gray* (London: Ward, Lock and Co, 1891), 275.

4. The Temperance Movement

Although the Victorian Era still saw narcotic consumers confronted with religious activists who propagated teetotalism in favour of the rejection of morally injurious drugs, their attitudes towards coca were an exception. Many of the anti-narcotic movements, such as the temperance movement, were motivated by religious beliefs and values since the time "was marked by a revival of religious activity unmatched since the day of the Puritans."[98] Nevertheless, while there was a strong Anti-Opium Movement that reached its peak with the founding of the Society for the Suppression of the Opium Trade, no such things happened for coca and cocaine. Every now and then, believers would make their voices heard in Parliament or in the media but there was hardly any opposition of them towards the novelty drugs which comes as a surprise. It is therefore even more necessary to investigate what role the temperance movement played in shaping public opinion on coca in addition to other social and cultural developments.

Originally, the temperance movement preached abstinence from all intoxicating substance and warned about their impact on society since, according to them, they posed a threat to moral degradation and public health. Prominent leaders such as Sir Joseph Pease, later president of Society for the Suppression of the Opium Trade (SSOT), also utilized their political influence to disseminate their beliefs, but surprisingly, the inclusion of cocaine was negligent. Nevertheless, religion "shaped that code of moral behavior [...] which we still call, rightly or wrongly, 'Victorianism'" wherefore their role in the career of coca mattered.[99]

The comparatively guarded reaction by fervent believers possibly stemmed from the previous change of mind of churchmen in South America in the sixteenth century. When the conquistadores forced Roman Catholicism upon the indigenous populations, Christianity posed a threat to the coca culture since the native coca habit was interpreted as an act of the devil and therefore regarded irreconcilable with religion. As a result, the Spaniards banned all coca until they realised it was a daily necessity that facilitated work in the mines. It did not take long until the Catholic church took a one-eighty turn and praised the drug for its miraculous properties, even suggesting it to be brought to

---

98 Josef F Altholz, "The Warfare of Conscience with Theology," The Victorian Web, accessed 18th June 2025, https://www.victorianweb.org/religion/altholz/a2.html.

99 Ibid.

Spain to sustain work of labourers there. Despite its inherent image as a heathenish cultural marker for the native population, coca's medicinal benefits eventually outweighed religious concerns which ensured its continuance.

Another reason for that exceptional attitude by believers was the circumstance that even after the discovery of cocaine and successively, its hypodermic application, the spread of the habit did not by far reach the same levels as the opium habit. This was due to a lack of accessibility, affordability, and availability for all social classes which prevented regular use and abuse. Ironically, this indicated that believers did not take an anti-narcotic stance because of a specific drug but made it dependent on whom it affected the most. In opium's case, physical and moral deterioration affected the working class in the home country and the seemingly poor, disadvantaged, and less civilised foreigner in the East. A coca or cocaine habit in both areas of society was almost unheard of in the Victorian Era to call for increased awareness and action. This means that believers opposed narcotics only – regardless of whether they had circulated for decades or were a novelty – if they viewed them as a danger to morality.

Among Victorian believers campaigning against intoxicants, one faith stood out: Quakerism. Having a Quaker faith in the Victorian Era often served as a motif for philanthropic activities, including the foundation of pharmaceutical companies. This circumstance is especially visible in the communication between Sturge and Thiselton-Dyer since Sturge's father, who also went by the first name Joseph, was a close friend of William Allen, the co-owner of Allen & Hanbury's, after 1792.[100] The families were tied by their religious background which is also reminiscent in the correspondence between Alfred Gravely Howard and Kew. Howard's grandfather was Quaker Luke Howard, who founded a pharmaceutical company with William Allen in 1798 that would later be renamed Howard & Sons after Allen had left.[101] It is therefore not surprising that the connection between Kew and pharmaceutical chemists was close from the very beginning and grew in importance simultaneously with coca's growing importance.

However, the narcotic and dangerous medicine they were selling in their pharmacies often interfered with their philanthropic goals. On the one hand, they wanted to contribute to improvements in public health, and on the other hand, rejecting to sell certain drugs on religious grounds would have proven

100 "Joseph Sturge," Quakers in the World, accessed 18th June 2025, https://www.quakersintheworld.org/quakers-in-action/285/Joseph-Sturge.

101 "Howard and Sons Limited {Chemists}," ACC/1037, The London Archives.

uneconomic since the public had a desire for them. In this business, they were walking a fine line that challenged their faith and entrepreneurial spirit at the same time. The Pharmaceutical Society argued as early as 1844 that "prohibition of their sale [i.e., poisons], even if practicable, would be attended with very serious commercial inconvenience."[102] As a result, pharmacists who were also Quakers or fervent believers hardly engaged in anti-narcotic movements, much in contrast to those in other professions. MPs Sir Wilfried Lawson, the Earl of Stanhope, Joseph Brotherton, Sir John Kennaway, and Alfred J Webb, for example, took a stance against the British opium trade and their colleague Sir Pease later presided over the SSOT. Their engagement received much attention but did not lead to major developments which might be a reason why there was no Anti-Coca or Anti-Cocaine Society, apart from the fact that the coca trade never reached the same extent.

5. Narcotics, Addiction, and Crime

The line between medicinal and recreational use of a drug was often a thin one – where did pain relief end and pleasure begin? Could a remedy that was praised as a mood elevator count as a sort of anti-depressant at that time or was it a means to fuel hedonistic tendencies? In any case, the continuous and increasing consumption of narcotics, particularly of opiates and cocaine, inevitably led to undesirable consequences both for the individual and society. Towards the end of the nineteenth century, characters such as Dorian Gray or Mr Hyde were not fictional anymore but represented the people who succumbed to their vice and posed a threat to society. The consumer became an addict whose cravings would sometimes lead him into immoral and unlawful behaviour that gave reason to worry and contributed to political regulations on the sale of narcotics.

"The vegetable kingdom has contributed its quota of substances noxious to life," wrote Arthur Griffins in 1899, "[...] and many of them have been associated with great crimes."[103] Unsurprisingly, poisonings ranged among the most prominent crimes associated with those substances but as Griffins continued, the regulations concerning the sale of poisons at the end of the century helped

102 "On the Sale of Poisons," *Pharmaceutical Journal* 4 (1844/5), 341.

103 Arthur Griffins, *Mysteries of Police and Crime. A General Survey of Wrongdoing and its Pursuit. Volume II* (London: Cassell and Company Ltd, 1899), 146, 147.

reduce their occurrence to a certain extent.[104] On the one hand, this concerned cases of self-poisoning, i.e., suicide, and on the other hand, it concerned the poisoning of others, often with the purpose of killing them. Whereas poisonings from opium remained prevalent due to its relatively easy and cheap procurement, cocaine poisonings were on the rise but remained less popular than morphine due to its limited affordability. It can be assumed that most of those were not intentional, especially when they occurred in a medicinal setting, but if outside the medicinally induced realm, consumers always risked overdoses without proper knowledge.

Historians Virginia Berridge and Griffith Edwards collected valuable numbers concerning the deaths from narcotics in Britain which reveals that an average of 5.3 people in a million died from narcotic consumption between 1863 and the end of the Victorian Era in 1901.[105] Of those 5.3, about 3.7 accounted for accidental deaths and 1.6 for accidental suicides from narcotics. In some years, a minute percentage accounted for wrongful deaths that were not accidental or that resulted from the execution of the death penalty. The primary narcotic causing death was opium and its preparation laudanum while cocaine was responsible for the death of up to 0.6 people in a million in 1901.[106]

Contemporary Griffins claimed that most male poisoners were "found among medical practitioners" who possessed "intimate knowledge [...] of the fatal properties of drugs" and could easily "cover up their tracks" but his examples posed singularities in the medical profession and did not include cocaine poisonings, for example.[107] Cocaine was not administered by a physician or surgeon for the intentional poisoning or killing of a patient – fatal doses were still widely unknown. If it did occur, the responsibility weighed heavy on a bona fide physician as in the case of a Russian doctor that committed suicide over the death of a patient whom he had given too high a dose of cocaine.[108] Medicine had progressed fast in the Victorian Era so that poisonings of any sort were not that easy disguise anymore and victims – or their relatives – could file lawsuits for improper administration, as previously explained.

This progress in medicine made it clear that poisoning was not necessarily a one-time incident but that continuous poisoning could also become an ill-

104 Griffins, *Mysteries of Police and Crime*, 157.

105 Berridge and Edwards, *Opium and the People*, Table 3.

106 Ibid., Table 4.

107 Griffins, *Mysteries of Police and Crime*, 136.

108 "-," *Dortmunder Zeitung* (6th December 1886), 6.

ness known as addiction. Berridge and Edwards claimed that "[t]he 'cocaine habit' was, through the connection with morphine, incorporated within the general disease view of addiction" and that "cocaine users seemed more of an autonomous, non-medical personality than the morphinist or opium addict."[109] But whereas the first part can generally be agreed with, due to increasing concern about treating the morphine habit with cocaine, the latter has little to do with the facts. Their assumption contradicts the fact that "autonomous, non-medical" personalities lacked the accessibility to cocaine for a long time – besides of questions of affordability – and by the time this changed at the end of the nineteenth century, restrictive regulations concerning its sales had already been put into place. In fact, it was the medical profession that first had accessed to cocaine and did not shy away from self-trials, as Freud's case has demonstrated.

The media picked up on this development in raising awareness with newspaper headlines such as "Suicide with Cocaine" or "The Supposed Death from Cocaine" that should illustrate that cocaine was equally as dangerous to public health as opium or morphine.[110] Firstly, this should inform people that cocaine was a powerful narcotic for which fatal doses were still widely unknown even among the medical profession, and secondly, this should elucidate the consequences of careless administration of cocaine at home. It also served the purpose of preventing recreational consumption that led to accidental deaths, as even consumption observed by a physician came with its uncertainties.

Despite of fictional characters such as Sherlock Holmes who evoked the impression that recreational use of cocaine was prevalent among non-medical people, this did not represent reality in Victorian Britain. Consumers of cocaine usually encountered the narcotic when it was medicinally recommended and prescribed by a physician. There was certainly a risk of difficulty of withdrawal which caused patients to take cocaine longer than necessary, but once again, this was a costly venture, especially when administered subcutaneously, so what we would call recreational use of cocaine could only affect a very limited circle of people. If anything, Berridge's and Edwards' argument makes more sense the other way round, that morphine and opium addicts were "autonomous, non-medical" personalities. Those two narcotics were available, af-

109 Berridge and Edwards, *Opium and the People*, 223.

110 "Suicide with Cocaine," *The Daily News* (9th April 1896), 2; "The Supposed Death from Cocaine," *The Daily News* (14th October 1896), 6.

fordable, and accessible so that consumers did not require medical attention or advice for their administration.

However, cocaine joined the ranks of prominent narcotics such as opium and morphine when it came to criticism regarding their threat to public health and morality. "The cocaine habit, more pernicious than the morphine neurosis, is the certain entailment of its frequent administration, and its thraldom is far more tyrannical than the slavery of opium," was Dr Hughes quoted in an article in the *Lancet*.[111] It entered the range of poisons that the public had to be protected from. As early as 1858, the Pharmaceutical Society stated: "The true and legitimate object of the poisons bill [was] to protect the public in England against injury arising from crime and carelessness in the use of dangerous drugs" and this accounted both for old narcotics and new ones on the market.[112] Neither coca, nor cocaine could become crowd-pleasers for Victorian society because their lifespan was limited by medicinal, social, and political circumstances. Although coca seemed a very promising novel narcotic that enjoyed popularity in several European countries between the 1860s and 1880s, it eventually had to succumb to the overwhelming negative consequences emerging from the abuse of its alkaloid.

111 Mattison, "Cocaine Dosage," 1025.

112 "Editorial," *Pharmaceutical Journal* 17 (1857/8), 201.

Chapter V: Restrictive Regulations

1. Relevance Today

In the face of the United Nations 66th session of the Commission on Narcotic Drugs in Vienna 2023, political debates surrounding the legalisation of coca were more present than ever. Coca-producing countries in the twenty-first century that are also concerned with illegal cocaine production such as Bolivia and Colombia utilised the conference to explain that coca leaf had wrongfully been put on an equal footing with cocaine and demanded not only a reversal of its illegalisation but also justice for decade-long discrimination of the whole coca culture in South America. An extract of the introductory speech given by Bolivia's vice president David Choquehuanca at the meeting is therefore worth quoting here in full:

> [...] la Convención sobre Estupefacientes ha cometido un error histórico, un atentado a la cultura de los pueblos originarios decretando que: "La Hoja de Coca esta condenada al exterminio en los próximos 25 anos". [...] los operadores de la geopolítica de dominación del occidente han intervenido su cultivo natural, su uso ritual y su consume tradicional, implementado programas de erradicación de la hoja de coca por los delitos que nunca ha cometido. [...] El sentido colonial de la retórica [...] ha demostrado incapacidad de aprender, transceder y reconducir el estado de consciencia unificada entre los Pueblos Originarios y la Sagrada Hoja de Coca. [...] Cuando los mecanismos y la normative son negligentes y no resilientes las políticas se tornan en una mentira. Cuando las leyes y el derecho son ineficientes la justicia es injusta, y se destruye a sí misma. Cuando cae la cortina de mentiras sobre la hoja de coca es momento de liberar la verdad y lograr que la humanidad la conozca. [...]

> La Libertad de la hoja de coca nadie nos va a regalar, la liberación se Conquista con acciones resilientes, trascendiendo las circunstancias adversas que enganan, que discriminant, que hacen sufrir. [...][1]

Choquehuanca's inflammatory speech greatly illustrated the meaning of coca for the indigenous population that has been so deeply embedded in South American culture, yet at the same time he blamed Western powers of wresting this valuable part of their history from them. Colonising and successively illegalising the coca leaf contributed to a distortion of the truth about its relevance in history, for medicine, and as nutrient which also violated the sovereignty of the countries from where it originated. He therefore demanded a decolonialisation of the coca leaf that does justice to the suffering experienced by the natives for centuries. It is his heartfelt wish that the "destrucción de la imagen del código de cultura de vida a escala mundial" comes to an end.[2] After his passionate defence of coca, Choquehuanca clarified that coca was incomparable to the illegal production of cocaine in his country and furthermore invited other countries to accompany the critical examination and a potential reclassification of coca listed in schedule one of illegal narcotics issued by the UN. In comparing both coca and cocaine, he picked up on the challenge people in nineteenth-century Britain faced when restrictions had been issued for the

1 David Choquehuanca, "Descolonizar la Hoja de Coca en el Tiempo de Pachakuti," United Nations 66th session of the Commission on Narcotic Drugs, Vienna, March 2023, accessed 18th June 2025, https://www.unodcol.org/documents/commissions/CND/CND_Sessions/CND_66/Item_3_-_Bolivia.pdf; transl.: "[...] the Convention on Narcotics has committed an historical error, an assault on the indigenous people who decree that: "The Coca leaf is doomed for extinction within the next 25 years". [...] the geopolitical agents of dominating Western powers have interfered with its natural cultivation, its ritual use, and its traditional consumption in implementing eradication programmes for the crimes the coca leaf has never committed. [...] Colonial notions in their rhetoric have demonstrated incapacity to understand, transcend, and redirect the unified state of consciousness between the indigenous people and the holy coca leaf. [...] When the mechanisms and the norms are neglected and fragile, politics turns into a lie. When the laws and the rights are ineffective, justice is unjust and it destroys itself. When the curtain of lies falls over the coca leaf, it is time to reveal the truth and get humanity to acknowledge it. [...] Nobody will give us the freedom of the coca leaf, the liberation is achieved by resilient actions that transcends adverse circumstances that deceive, discriminate and cause harm. [...]."

2 Ibid., transl.: "destruction of the image of the cultural code of life on a global scale."

first time and he showed how this challenge had persisted for more than a century.

During the conference, this distinction between coca and cocaine was also highlighted by Colombia that assumed the most prominent role as the top producer of cocaine on the global market in 2023. Vice minister Laura Gabriela Gil Savastano explained that her country was tired of the war on drugs because it had worsened living conditions for the Colombian population and caused thousands of deaths: "Colombia está cansada. [...] Por más de 50 anos, mi país ha abanderado la lucha contra el problema mundial de las Drogas [...]."[3] Nevertheless, she agreed with Bolivia that including coca as a controlled substance was "un error histórico contra los pueblos autócọnos de Los Andes. La planta no es el problema; la planta es parte de nuestra historia y nuestras tradiciones."[4] Savastano also called upon the countries with the biggest consumer markets of cocaine who, in her opinion, have not done their share in preventing the spread of illegal narcotics.

Despite being less passionate about the re-legalisation of coca than Bolivia, Savastano's support in the face of the overwhelming war on drugs in her country was remarkable. Even more so, since the mother country of the 'sacred plant of the Inca' took a rather different stance. In contrast to its neighbours Bolivia and Colombia, the president of the national commission on drug control in Peru, Emilio Arce de la Torre Bueno, refrained from calling the illegalisation of coca a historical mistake and merely "reconoce el valor ancestral, tradicional y cultural de la hoja de coca de origen lícito, cuyas áreas de cultivo se encuentran devidamente delimitadas y reglamantadas."[5] He made it clear that coca's

3 S E Laura Gabriela Gil Savastano, "Debate General," United Nations 66th session of the Commission on Narcotic Drugs, Vienna, March 2023, accessed 18th June 2025, https://www.unodcol.org/documents/commissions/CND/CND_Sessions/CND_66/Item_3_-_Colombia.pdf, transl.: "Colombia is tired. [...] For over 50 years, my country has led the fight against the global drug problem [...]."

4 Savastano, "Debate General," transl.: "a historical error against the indigenous people of the Andes. The plant is not the problem; the plant is part of our history and our traditions."

5 Emilio Arce de la Torre Bueno, "Discurso del Presidente Ejecutivo de Devida, en la Sesion plenaria CND," United Nations 66th session of the Commission on Narcotic Drugs, Vienna, March 2023, accessed 18th June 2025, https://www.unodcol.org/documents/commissions/CND/CND_Sessions/CND_66/Item_3_-_Peru.pdf; transl.: "recognises the ancestral, traditional, and cultural value of the coca leaf of lawful origin, whose areas of cultivation find themselves deviously limited and regulated."

role as a raw material for the manufacture of cocaine was of more importance than its significance for the native population. Torre Bueno was convinced that increased coca production would lure vulnerable families into illicit drug production which would endanger the country's economy as a whole. Therefore, the best strategy was to concur with the UN's recommendations concerning drug control.

Eventually, Bolivia succeeded with its plea in 2024, when

> "[...] después de más de seis décadas de injusticia, persecución, amenazas, violación de derechos y un silencio cómplice, Bolivia reclama a la Organización Mundial de la Salud un Examen Critico Científico basado en cuatro criterios: farmacológico, toxicológico, terapéutico tradicional y epidemiológico, para sacar a la luz la verdad científica, verdad que nuestros pueblos y tradiciones saben desde los milenios."[6]

This critical examination of the coca leaf was also endorsed by Colombia, stating that they trust "[...] que el studio científico [of the WHO, KE] [...] nos dará la razón, y que esta Comisión [i.e., the UNODC, KE] también escuchará a la ciencia."[7] The examination was still ongoing in summer 2025 and a voting on the matter is expected to conclude at the 2026 conference.[8]

---

6 David Choquehuanca, "Palabras Inaugurales," United Nations 68th session of the Commission on Narcotic Drugs, Vienna, March 2025, accessed 20th August 2025, https://estatements.unmeetings.org/estatements/31.0365/20250310100000000/KntrDKxQ/DMIoUx-kUIW_vna_es.pdf; transl.: "[...] after more than six decades of injustice, persecution, threats, violation of rights and complicit silence, Bolivia demands that the World Health Organization carries out a scientific critical examination based on four criteria: pharmacological, toxicological, traditional therapeutic and epidemiological, to bring to light the scientific truth, a truth that our peoples and traditions have known for millennia."

7 Laura Sarabia, "Intervención Debate General," United Nations 68th session of the Commission on Narcotic Drugs, Vienna, March 2025, accessed 20th August 2025, https://estatements.unmeetings.org/estatements/31.0365/20250310100000000/KntrDKxQ/PIVEb-KEr_vna_es.pdf; transl.: "[...] that the scientific study will prove us right and that this Commission will also listen to science."

8 A supporting dossier on behalf of Bolivia can be found here: Government of Bolivia, "World Health Organization Critical Review of the Coca Leaf Supporting Dossier," accessed 20th August 2025, https://hojadecoca.cancilleria.gob.bo/wp-content/uploads/2023/09/Coca-Review-Dossier-Annex-English-revised-VP-240523.pdf.

The speeches of these three countries – Bolivia, Colombia, and Peru – reflected questions that the world and Britain already had to deal with when coca first came up in the International Opium Commission in 1909. On the one hand, they asked for the distinction between the raw material and the purified product in a medicinal aspect and on the other hand, they asked about the economic and social consequences of possible restrictions. However, the Victorian debate on coca did not include its role as a cultural marker for the native populations (due to colonial and supremacist currents at that time). It is therefore necessary to revisit the decades leading up to the International Opium Convention 1912 to understand the initial motifs and processes that led to the inclusion of coca, cocaine, and preparations thereof as internationally controlled substances.

2 From Medicinal Marvel to Political Menace

The last stage of the career cycle of coca was concerned with political restrictions and regulations. In Victorian times, this affected restrictions both within the home country and in the British colonies around the globe. Coca's exceptionality as a narcotic in this regard stemmed from the challenge for politicians to distinguish between the raw and purified product in their decision-making. Whereas for opium and morphine, the effects were pretty obvious as they were widespread and visible, coca consumers displayed no or hardly any symptoms of addiction that could spark concerns. Cocaine consumption, on the contrary, had detrimental effects if used inappropriately and such reports interfered with those on the drug's medicinal benefits. Consequently, this development prompted politicians to paint both the original plant and the potent manufactured narcotic with the same brush in declaring both 'poisons' in the 1908 Poisons and Pharmacy Act in Britain.

Coca also posed an exception in a political aspect since it was a drug non-native to the British Empire which exacerbated restrictions. When British-grown opium was forced onto China, it was no problem for Britain to disregard China's regulations. But when the situation was reversed and other countries imported a foreign drug into the empire, it became more difficult for Britain to take action and it required a different strategy. In India, for example, there were laws in place to regulate opium sales and consumption but initially, they did not include other narcotics such as coca and cocaine. It was also almost impossible to determine the amount of cocaine being imported into the colony since shipments continued to be mislabelled, both intentionally and unintentionally.

While it did not necessarily concern coca, criticism of cocaine arose from three key areas that fuelled political restrictions as a final step. At the beginning stood the medical community that increasingly expressed reservations about its use when side effects and accidental poisoning revealed the risks of cocaine consumption. In addition, the emergence of the concept of addiction as explained in Chapter IV put both coca and cocaine into the same category of narcotics as opium and morphine, even if the former was significantly lagging behind in potency. These circumstances could not be disguised, so that many politicians and medical men soon started criticising the addictive and morally deteriorating effects of cocaine consumption. Especially the temperance movement, newspapers, and authors of fiction regarded it their responsibility to highlight its vicious consequences that contributed to societal ills. As this criticism became more apparent, political circles became aware of cocaine's potential for abuse and harm to society and eventually realised the need for legal action to restrict its availability on the British market. The combination of medical, social, and moral concerns about cocaine's impact on individuals and society thus formed the prelude that contributed to the legal regulation of both coca and cocaine.

Legislative action against the cultivation, trade, and consumption of narcotics in Britain took a long time which exacerbated their containment. New legislation had to be debated in both houses of Parliament and voted on before a Bill was passed that would eventually turn into an Act or an amendment thereof. There were constant delays due to the houses waiting on so-called expert opinions, especially in the House of Lords, and politicians lacking support in the House to take action in one way or another. From the idea to the implementation of a new law roughly two years passed. This was equally true for parliamentary publications such as the Opium Report which took almost twenty-two months from when an investigation into the matter was first debated in June 1893 to its publication in April 1895. Acts improving public health and restricting the accessibility and availability of narcotics were no different which hampered quick action.

When coca underwent the medicinal and pharmaceutical phase, it already became apparent that the distinction between the original plant, coca, and its potent alkaloid cocaine was not as easy as anticipated today. The determination of which one posed an actual threat to public health was thus exacerbated and raised the question if there was a possibility for recreational use for one of the two that did not have the potential to cause addiction. From a modern point of view, we know that cocaine has a high addictive potential wherefore it is classified as a narcotic in most countries and can only be used for limited medicinal purposes.[9] For coca, the potential to cause addiction has remained unclear, back in the Victorian Era as today. Even in the twenty-first century, South American countries are still fighting for the removal of coca off the list of narcotics, as there is no evidence that can confirm that coca tea, for example, can cause addiction.[10]

As the criticism of narcotics in general increased around mid-century, pharmacists demanded political action to restrict their sales. This did not yet affect cocaine but primarily the go-to panacea opium, its derivate morphine, and other narcotics. Until then, all of these were freely available over the counter without any system to check the amount being sold to individuals which meant that customers could go to different pharmacies and accumulate a stock for themselves. As a result, narcotics were often overdosed and caused poisonings but they were also abused to commit suicide: "16,000 people engaged in the sale of poisons [...] [and] [t]here were 500 cases every year of deaths from poisoning, either intentional or unintentional [...]."[11] Parliament therefore requested the examination of the issue by a board of qualified professionals from the Pharmaceutical Society, the College of Physicians, and the Society of Apothecaries.[12] Despite a few differences in opinion between the three examining parties and the aforementioned lengthy legislative process,

---

9 Ophthalmologists are allowed to prescribe low percentage cocaine solution in illnesses of the eye. Similar to opium, whose derivates, such as morphine, are also used in surgery and pain management, the marvellous properties of the plant did not disappear with the arrival of their illegal recreational use, "Kokain und Crack: Drogenprofil," European Union Drugs Agency, accessed 18th June 2025, https://www.euda.europa.eu/publications/drug-profiles/cocaine_de.

10 Keep in mind that the cocaine content in coca leaves amounts to around 0.5% and that oral consumption avoids the first-pass effect, meaning that the liver absorbs most of the narcotic before it reaches its target, "Routes of drug administration," WikiLectures, accessed 18th June 2025, https://www.wikilectures.eu/index.php?title=Routes_of_drug_administration&oldid=25063.

11 HL Deb 4th June 1857 vol. 145 col. 1093.

12 HL Deb 4th June 1858 vol. 150 col. 1509.

parliament got an act underway that would put the sales of narcotics under stricter regulations.[13] This act became known as the Pharmacy Act 1868.

The act was a consequence of sociocultural and medicinal developments of the previous decades. Firstly, there was rising concern over public health during a time when the sale of medicine was unregulated of which some turned out potentially harmful with the advances in medical science.[14] At the same time, the pharmaceutical profession was established as one that required appropriate testing and examinations to distinguish qualified pharmacists from so-called quack doctors. Therefore, the Pharmaceutical Society, founded in 1841, was implemented as the formal agency to keep a register on qualified chemists and druggists to ensure that medicines were only issued by knowledgeable professionals.[15] This posed an important contribution to the safety and efficacy of drugs being sold, but poisons could still be sold over the counter, nonetheless, thus making further regulations necessary.

The Pharmacy Act coming into effect on 1st January 1869 was the most significant act concerning the regulations of poisons in the Victorian Era. For the first time, poisons had to be labelled as such and those dispensing poisons had to be qualified, registered, and needed to keep records of the sales and customers of poisons.[16] It also limited "the supplying of medicines by a medical man to his patients" which shifted the responsibility for the dispense of poisons to pharmacies to make it more controllable.[17] There were two parts in the act that listed poisonous substances, such as opium and all preparations thereof, but coca and cocaine were not yet part of this list. This did not come as a surprise as cocaine had just been discovered a few years prior, knowledge about its poisonous properties was still in its infancy, and the circumstance of it being hardly affordable for the average customer. Not only did the act improve the safety of public health through the distribution of dangerous substances only by trained professionals, but it also laid the groundwork for modern pharmaceutical regulation and subsequently influenced future drug regulations.

---

13 Berridge and Edwards, *Opium and the People*, 114, 115; Anne-Marie Coles, "Non-Linear Discourse and Control of Technology: The Pharmaceutical Society and Poisons Legislation in 19th-Century Britain," *Sociology* 51 (3) (2017), 520.

14 Holloway, *Royal Pharmaceutical Society of Great Britain, 1841–1991*, 150, 151.

15 Ibid., 96.

16 "The Pharmacy Act of 1868," *The Lancet* (14th November 1868), 649.

17 Ibid., 650.

Initially, it seemed as if the Pharmacy Act of 1868 proved effective since mortality rates from narcotics dropped significantly within the following two years.[18] However, they increased steadily until the end of the Victorian Era when mortality rates reached a peak that exceeded those numbers before the issuance of the act. Interestingly, this development only accounted for narcotic deaths of adults over the age of 20. In 1868, England registered 62 deaths in children and teenagers that dropped to 20 in 1890.[19] In the same time frame, narcotic deaths in adults increased from 78 to 144. Why was that? The problem was that the pharmacy act did recognise narcotics as drugs that had to subject to regulations but that those regulations were not intervening enough. Consumers could still obtain narcotics, now from licensed pharmacists instead from any street dealer and there were no limits as to its possession. In addition, prescriptions were kept by patients and could be filled by as many pharmacies as one liked. The decreasing mortality in narcotic deaths of children therefore rather stemmed from improved living conditions than the act alone but it became clear that further regulations were necessary to restrict the sale of poisons.

The forty years between the Pharmacy Act 1868 and the Poisons and Pharmacy Act 1908 were marked by a noteworthy absence of legislature concerning narcotics. A few circumstances have contributed to that. It is possible that politicians and the pharmaceutical profession regarded the Pharmacy Act as sufficient for the time and wanted to assess its impact over the following years. In addition, public health concerns shifted to other topics such as sanitation and housing conditions that required immediate action. This is visible in the Public Health Acts of 1872, 1875, 1878, 1891, 1897, and 1901. Nevertheless, the discovery of new poisons such as cocaine and an increased understanding of toxicology highlighted gaps in the Pharmacy Act 1868 that required additional regulations after the turn of the century.

In order to issue additional regulations on specific drugs, British politicians faced the challenge of defining what constituted a poison in the first place. This problem had already been identified in 1856 with professionals in the medical field debating the question in *The Times*. F E P rightfully asked "What is a poison?" and proposed that "[...] the law must either give a list of the poisons to which it applies [...] or it must give a definition of what a poison is, and leave it to the discretion of the retailer to decide what drugs fall under the

---

18 Berridge and Edwards, *Opium and the People*, Table 3.

19 Ibid., Table 4.

category."[20] However, the author thought the latter proceeding "to be unfair, obnoxious, and most inexpedient."[21] This was objected by another author given that a legal definition could already be found in "the 1st Victoria, chap. 85, sect. 2" which declared "[a]ny "destructive thing" which shall be criminally administered or taken by any person, and which by its nature and mode of operation shall destroy life, [is] legally a poison."[22] However, this definition was too narrowly considered as many substances were conducive and beneficial to one's health if taken in moderation and only deadly when taken in excess.

It does therefore not come as a surprise that politicians indeed preferred to provide a list they considered poisons rather than a more detailed definition, as the Pharmacy Act 1868 showed: "[...] several Articles named or described in the Schedule (A.) shall be deemed to be Poisons [...]."[23] Coca and cocaine, for example, were not yet part of this schedule and therefore not considered poisons. On the one hand, this facilitated the dispensing of poisons by pharmacists because they could rely on a specific list, but on the on the other hand, refraining from negotiating their definition and from putting it down in writing exacerbated further regulations.

Instead, a committee was founded after the turn of the century to investigate the effect of new drugs which provided a starting point for stricter regulations thereof. The investigation compromised any drug possibly detrimental to public health, including narcotics, wherefore they were generally labelled as poisons. In 1903, the Committee of Poisons published a list of deaths from poisons in England and Wales in 1899 but their list did not include any deaths from the wrongful use of cocaine for an estimated population of 32 million at that time.[24] However, it listed 97 deaths from other anaesthetics such as chlo-

---

20 F E P, "Sale of Poisons.," *The Times*, 22nd September 1856.

21 Ibid.

22 W W, "Sale of Poisons.," *The Times*, 10th October 1856.

23 *A Collection of the Public General Statutes Passed in the Thirty-First and Thirty-Second Years of the Reign of Her Majesty Queen Victoria: Being the Third Session of the Nineteenth Parliament of the United Kingdom of Great Britain and Ireland* (London: Eyre & Spottiswoode, 1868), 589.

24 House of Commons, *Report, Supplementary Report, and Minority Report of the Departmental Committee appointed by the Lord President of the Council to consider Schedule A. to the Pharmacy Act, 1868, to report the alterations therein which they deem expedient, and whether a Third Part should be added thereto, with a copy of the Minutes appointing the Committee, and a List of Witnesses examined. Pt. I (Pharmacy and Poisons: Sale of Poisons)*, Herbert Eustace Maxwell, 6th Baron Monreith (London: Wyman & Sons, 1903), 132.

roform and ether while opium and its derivates accounted for 76 accidental deaths and 69 suicides.[25] Although this list did not give reason to worry, the committee still advised that preparations of cocaine "should be added to [Part II of] Schedule A. of the Pharmacy Act, 1868" and that "it may be deemed desirable to specifically name [cocaine and morphine]" in Part I of said schedule.[26] This development was over 35 years in the making and despite cocaine poisoning not seeming reason to worry as a cause of death, the pharmaceutical industry and politics were well aware that cocaine was a poison, nonetheless.

Although the Committee of Poisons urged for the inclusion of cocaine in 1903, it took another five years until it was actually put into practice with the Poisons and Pharmacy Act of 1908. In the years in between, the Houses of Lords briefly debated the inclusion or exclusion of certain poisons and the correct wording thereof. They agreed that not only cocaine and its salts but also coca had to be added to the schedule with a small distinction in preparations that contained between 0.1% and 1% of the alkaloid (Part II) and those that contained more than 1% (Part I).[27] This meant that literally everything being prepared from coca leaves was put under restriction and needed to be labelled "with the name of the substance and the word 'Poisonous,' and with the name and address of the seller of the substance."[28] The act then came into effect after 1st January 1909.

Whereas the act distinguished between different kinds of poppies and their use (*papaver somniferum* which was restricted and *papaver rhoeas* which was not), coca did not deserve a closer look as to its poisonous content. There also existed different kinds of coca, e.g. *erythroxylum coca* or *erythroxylum novogranatense*, and they could all be used to produce cocaine to different extents, but the closer look concerned more the raw and purified product. At that time, Britain was not the only country that struggled with the distinction between coca and cocaine. France had similar reservations about coca when they were suddenly confronted with the addictive nature of its alkaloid. Previously giving rise to the father of coca wines, Angelo Mariani, France decided to take his *Vin* off the French Pharmaceutical Codex in 1910 after it had been listed there for more than 15 years. The meeting of the International Opium Commission

25 Ibid., 132, 133.

26 House of Commons, *Report, Supplementary Report, and Minority Report*, 135.

27 HL Deb 5th April 1906, vol. 155 col. 632; HL Deb 14th July 1908, vol. 192 col. 569.

28 "Poisons and Pharmacy Act, 1908," *Supplement to the British Medical Journal* (9th January 1909), 15, 16.

in Shanghai 1909 certainly cast a shadow over coca and caused France to be proactive about both the original plant and its alkaloid.

The debate about the difference in potency of the original plant coca and its alkaloid cocaine that occurred in pharmaceutical circles and public media in Britain did not enter parliament as it did for poppy varieties. This is surprising. It seems as if ignorance was not a motif for parliament to investigate the matter further and neither did coca's role as a cultural marker for the indigenous population play a role in that. The more likely explanation was that legislation against narcotics took too long and the pressure for Britain to issue stricter regulations was high. Teetotallers and supporters of the temperance movement in parliament had tried to restrict the sale of poisons for decades, as MP Theodore Taylor pointed out: "[...] [T]he real question at issue is not that of one dangerous drug only, but that all dangerous drugs should be under strict medical supervision."[29] In addition, the pressure from other countries, especially from the United States, forced Britain not to waste time on obtaining information from experts on the topic to make a deliberate decision.[30] A condemnation of all narcotics, regardless of their potency, did also not leave any loopholes that required future amendments of the law. But in doing so, Britain contributed to the successive debate that persisted until the United Nations 68th session of the Commission on Narcotic Drugs in Vienna 2025: Should coca and cocaine be painted with the same brush?

3. Politicising Cocaine

Cocaine did not occupy the minds of British politicians for a long time and debates on it turning into a severe threat to public health were non-existent until the International Opium Conference 1912. Even when the drug was mentioned, it was limited to just a few observations that can be considered negligent in comparison to the extensive debates on opium that spanned over a century. The comparably limited number of consumers of cocaine, insufficient knowledge about its toxicology, and the evolution of the concept of addiction at the

29 HC Deb, 27th June 1912, col. 594.

30 Compare Sir Joseph Pease: "[O]ur American friends are beginning to find out that the use of this drug [opium, KE] [...] is demoralizing to their people, and they have already passed a statute on the subject. [...] [I]n America, they find that this drug is as evil in its effects as in China," HC Deb 3rd April 1883 col. 1343.

end of the nineteenth century that affected all narcotics delayed debates. Cocaine was first brought up in the House of Commons in May 1901 when the Secretary of State for India, Lord G Hamilton, was asked about the apparent increasing cocaine consumption in India which he denied.[31] In a similar instance five years later, the Secretary of State for India, then a Mr John Morley, reassured the audience that "[t]he traffic in the drug has already been placed under restrictions in provinces where there was evidence of extensive and improper use" and that "in Delhi the habit is not at all widespread."[32] In the House of Lords, the consumption of cocaine in India never came up but they discussed the right termination of coca and preparations of its alkaloid for the inclusion in the Poisons and Pharmacy Bill 1909.[33]

The inclusion of cocaine in the International Opium Convention was mentioned only once shortly after it took place and it put an emphasis on preventing the spread of the habit in Asia rather than preventing the spread everywhere. The Marquess of Crewe explained that "it was a great deal to ask a country on humanitarian grounds to check the export of a drug of that kind [i.e., opium, KE] if there remained an unrestricted import from other sources of a worse drug or worse forms of the same drug – that is to say, such products as morphia and cocaine – into the very countries from which opium is being barred."[34] But for whom was it a great deal on humanitarian grounds? It is doubtful that India regarded it a challenge to limit exports or imports of any kind of drug on humanitarian grounds since they had witnessed the spread of the habit and the detrimental effects on its population by first-hand experience. They were the first ones to issue restrictions on opium in the empire, so they were obviously convinced of subsequent humanitarian benefits. Less drugs meant less consumption and better control which made the spread of addiction more manageable.

So, was the limitation of narcotic imports a big deal for Britain? By supporting the restriction of all types of narcotics in the colony, Britain clearly directed their policy on cocaine as being specific to India, rather than applying it uniformly to the whole Empire. But in fact, taking a turn on narcotic imports and exports on humanitarian grounds was a great deal for Britain itself rather than

31 HC Deb 13th May 1901, col. 1456–1457.

32 HC Deb 19th July 1906, col. 379.

33 HL Deb 14th July 1908, col. 569–571.

34 HL Deb 14th February 1912, col. 41.

for its colony. For the first time, the country had to accept the fact that humanitarian reasons in the global drug trade weighed more than financial interests which resulted from international pressure on behalf of other highly influential nations. Pioneer here was certainly the United States who issued the Drug Importation Act as early as 1848 to ensure specific strength and purity standards for narcotics which posed one of the earliest federal efforts to do so.[35] British supremacy caused a dilemma here between humanitarian and financial interests. This could only be resolved by drawing attention to the country supporting the fight against narcotics of the allegedly inferior Indian population. This smart move contributed to Britain not appearing as a selfish player in the drug business to keep its revenue, nor did it appear as an aggressor to Germany's profitable cocaine business. Instead, Britain emerged as the benefactor to the Asian people.

This is supported by the Marquess of Crewe's statement which illustrated that Parliament suddenly considered cocaine a worse narcotic than opium: "The unrestricted use of opium is undoubtedly a bad thing, but the unrestricted use of morphia and cocaine is very much worse [...]."[36] Although there had not been any relevant reports on the spread of the cocaine habit in Britain, the focus of attention was India where the drug was on the rise and caused public health concerns such as the opium habit a few decades earlier. There was in fact an ongoing investigation from the Cocaine Committee in India and Ceylon to investigate the matter but it took until summer 1912 that their final report was forwarded to the colonial secretary. The committee found that there was some illegitimate use and smuggling in both Ceylon and India but also, that there were strict regulations in place that encompassed the cultivation of coca, as well as limits concerning the possession and sales of cocaine.[37] The Marquess of Crewe must have therefore spoken about India in his role as Secretary of State there rather than reflecting on the current status of a cocaine addiction in the British people.

35 US Congress, *Congressional Record*, 30th Congress, 1st Session, 1848, Chapter 70, 237–239, accessed 18th June 2025, https://maint.locol.gov/law/help/statutes-at-large/30th-congress/session-1/c30s1ch70.pdf; Wesley J Heath, "America's First Drug Regulation Regime: The Rise and Fall of the Import Drug Act of 1848," *Food and Drug Law Journal* 59, no. 1 (2004), 170.

36 HL Deb 14th February 1912, col. 41.

37 Cocaine Committee, "Opium, Morphia, and Cocaine," 1–4.

4. The Role of Cocaine in India

Although the Indian princely states had already issued restrictions concerning narcotic consumption in their territories, Britain did not shy away to import cocaine into the country after 1903.[38] The first 40 kg valuing about £1,200 made it to British India in 1903 and within about two years, imports almost quadrupled so that in 1904–5 cocaine imports already matched that of opium, both amounting to 154 kg and 157 kg, respectively.[39] Although Merck of Darmstadt was the primary manufacturer of cocaine imports, Burgoyne's, Burrough's, and other British companies were part of the business as well which caused the value of cocaine to drop while the value of opium remained steady.[40] The Under Secretary of State for India argued that in some places like Calcutta, cocaine already substituted opium which gave reason to worry.[41]

As a consequence, the Indian Excise Committee then included cocaine and preparations thereof as "intoxicating drug[s]" in 1906, although opium was not part of that list.[42] The regulations concerning the sale of intoxicating drugs in India were more strictly enforced in areas where a possibly increasing habit became apparent but in successive years, such restrictions led to increased smuggling. P R Cadell, the collector of customs in Bombay, reported in April 1907 that "cocaine [was] being smuggled to a very considerable extent" and that "checking its importation" came with great difficulty in his province wherefore he urged the commissioner of customs to enquire about the situation in other

38 After the British government took over control of India from the East India Company, about half of the territory was ruled by viceroys in British provinces while the other half were princely states. They were governed by an Indian ruler which constituted a form of indirect rule, see Barbara Ramusack, *The Indian Princes and their States* (Cambridge: Cambridge University Press, 2004), 85, 87.

39 *Tables Relating to the Trade of British India with British Possessions and Foreign Countries 1900–01 to 1904–05* (London: Wyman and Sons, 1906), 48; *Tables Relating to the Trade of British India with British Possessions and Foreign Countries 1901–02 to 1905–06* (London: Wyman and Sons, 1907),14.

40 *Tables Relating to the Trade of British India 1901–02 to 1905–06*, 15; Cocaine was worth up to 15 times more than opium; *Tables Relating to the Trade of British India with British Possessions and Foreign Countries 1904–5 to 1908–9* (London: Eyre and Spottiswoode, 1910),11.

41 House of Commons, *Statement exhibiting the Moral and Material Progress and Condition of India during the Year 1902–03* (London: Eyre and Spottiswoode, 1904), 82.

42 *Report of the Indian Excise Committee, 1905–06* (London: Darling & Son, 1907), 2, 137;House of Commons, *Statement exhibiting the Moral and Material Progress and Condition of India during the Year 1900–01* (London: Eyre and Spottiswoode, 1902), 92.

provinces as well.[43] The enquiry concluding nine months later then found that besides of Bombay, only the cities of Ahmedabad and Surat seemed to have a problem with the spread of a cocaine habit due to extensive smuggling of the drug. The commissioner therefore recommended that the collectors in those cities kept a closer eye on incoming parcels from England and Germany but that seemed insufficient given that the cocaine habit was on the rise.

Realising the limitations of these measurements Sir Edward Norman Baker, Lieutenant-Governor of Bengal, thus proposed an amendment of the United Provinces Excise Act of 1896. Baker remarked that "the consumption of cocaine [was] very much on the increase and that the spread of the habit constitute[d] a serious danger" wherefore the objective was to enable "strict control [in all of India, KE] which that law allow[ed] in respect of persons licensed to sell it and in regard to the amount which buyers may possess."[44] After hearing several members of the Indian Legislative Council on the matter, the bill was passed in 1906 without any objections. As Maharaja Sir Mohammad Ali Mohammad Khan stated:

> [...] [I]t is the duty of the Government as well as the people to save the ignorant masses from the injurious effects of the poisonous drug. It is in the fitness of things that the use and possession of such obnoxious and dangerous drugs should be prohibited and made penal. Such legislation is in itself a proof of the sympathy and regard which the benign Government has for the well-being of the people.[45]

Although the Indian government seemed to have had the right intention in limiting the importation and sales of cocaine in the colony, smuggling existed to a greater extent than they had assumed. This was the primary reason why prices dropped significantly from about £73 per ounce of cocaine in 1905 to £45 in 1908.[46] The ineffectiveness of the amended law was visible in successive years

43 Government of India, Revenue Department, "Accompaniments to Government Resolution," dated 3rd July 1908, No. 6666, Appendix A.

44 Government of India, Legislative Department, "Annexure to Bill to amend the Excise Act, 1896."

45 Government of India, "Extract from the Abstract of Proceedings of Council, dated 8th November 1905. The United Provinces Excise Law Amendment Bill, 1905."

46 *Tables Relating to the Trade of British India 1904–5 to 1908–9*, 11; *Tables Relating to the Trade of British India with British Possessions and Foreign Countries 1905–6 to 1909–10* (London: Eyre and Spottiswoode, 1911), 33.

when consuls reported that in the province of Burma alone roughly 37 kg of cocaine were seized in 1910 which made up over two thirds of the total of legal cocaine exports in the same year.[47] These developments in India raised concerns in the House of Commons who worried that the cocaine habit spread there as quickly as the opium habit a few decades earlier.[48]

The governors of the provinces still seemed oblivious or naïve to observe this development. To further investigate the matter, a Cocaine Committee formed in 1912 and revealed more about the process of restrictions and the parties involved in India, Ceylon, and the Straits Settlement in a formerly classified document on opium, morphine (formerly called morphia), and cocaine. According to H L Dowbiggin, acting Inspector-General of Police, no cocaine habit existed in the Provinces and in Ceylon, the habit was limited to "moormen and prostitutes" who used it as an aphrodisiac.[49] The number of wholesalers and medical practitioners in Ceylon was limited to four and two, respectively, and numbers for the rest of British India were also comparatively low.[50] Those who prescribed cocaine had to be medical practitioners and those who sold it needed to hold a license to do so while occasionally, the police registered names of customers who purchased the narcotic.[51]

Nevertheless, Dowbiggin reported that the "sale ha[d] increased 400 per cent. since 1908" which required additional measures.[52] Apparently, Ceylon and Burma had the strictest regulations in place concerning cocaine, and morphia, under which patients were only allowed to request one refill of the drug that could not exceed a maximum quantity. Even so, the committee issued recommendations to lower this maximum quantity since it left a loophole to stock cocaine by purchasing it from different pharmacists and furthermore urged the Indian government to restrict the importation and sale of syringes for hypodermic injections.[53] Making those recommendations indicated a close observation of the spread of the habit and a thorough understanding of proper measures that could put a check on cocaine.

47 *Review of the Trade of India in 1909–10* (London: Wyman & Sons, 1911), 23.

48 HC 29th July 1906, col. 379.

49 Cocaine Committee, "Opium, Morphia, and Cocaine," 7.

50 Ibid., 2.

51 Ibid., 7, 8.

52 Ibid., 8.

53 Ibid., 3, 4.

In addition, the report listed over a dozen European manufacturers and importers of coca and cocaine that served the Indian market, including E Merck & Co. of Darmstadt as the "biggest manufacturers in the world."[54] Surprisingly, all of them were German and not a single principal manufacturer or dealer was British. This stood in sharp contrast to reports by the Revenue Department in India four years prior that had listed British companies Burrough's & Wellcome, Burgoyne & Burbidge, and Lormer & Co. This either points towards German exceeding British pharmaceutical companies in importing cocaine to India or towards the British withdrawing from the trade altogether. The former explanation seems more likely. Despite stricter regulations on cocaine imports, it appears as if Germany took over the field and made the British share negligible which was also visible in increased seizures of cocaine from Merck that was smuggled into the country.

The report of the Cocaine Committee showed that the British colonies had much stricter regulations in place and that they were issued earlier than in the motherland. As early as 1903, importing cocaine into India and selling it for other than medicinal purposes was forbidden in several provinces although it was not yet declared an intoxicating substance or poison until 1906. In England, cocaine was only listed as a poison in 1908 when it became subject to the same rule of being available solely for medicinal purposes. However, many provinces in India also limited the quantity that could be stocked and dispensed by vendors which was not regulated in England. In Ceylon, for example, licensed druggists and medical practitioners could not sell or buy more than one ounce of cocaine while private consumers were only allowed a maximum of 6 grains of powder or 10 grains in a solution.[55] Historian James Mills has argued that stricter control of cocaine in India might have stemmed from increasing concerns for "Indian youth and Indian women" but the aforementioned accessibility and availability at that time contradict

54 Cocaine Committee, "Opium, Morphia, and Cocaine," 7; other manufacturers included C. F. Bohringer, Soehne, C. H. Bohringer, Soehne, Knoll & Co., T. L. Geyer, Zemmer & Co., Frieder Witte, John Didler Beiber, Chemische Fabrick auf Actien e Shewing, J. D. Reidel, Sehe & Co, in addition to importers Cargills, Bohringer, Colombo Apothecaries Co., and International Stores.

55 Cocaine Committee, "Opium, Morphia, and Cocaine," 3; in grams: 0.39 and 0.65, respectively.

this claim.[56] The reason the Maharaja gave for the regulations in his country, "to save the ignorant masses," also appeared far-fetched – we have already established that neither coca nor cocaine were narcotics for the masses. However, accessibility and availability of cocaine was much more limited there and Britain still regarded India as an inferior country where stricter regulations on drugs were necessary, particularly with opium as a prelude.[57] In any way, those regulations were a step into the right direction to prevent harm to public health by narcotics.

Some historians argue that by imposing stricter regulations in the colony in comparison to the home country, Britain was outsourcing a problem. In doing so, the responsibility to handle the growing concern over cocaine addiction was shifted to the British Indian government who would also have to face potential criticism should their measures fail. On the one hand, this might be true as Britain only introduced regulations concerning coca and cocaine – among other so-called poisons – in 1909, as explained above. This would have given them sufficient time to wait and assess how effective the measures were in British India to develop appropriate domestic restrictions later on. On the other hand, the spread of the cocaine habit in British India was partly self-created as Britain was the primary importer of the drug in the first years of the twentieth century.[58] The demographic situation in the colony and the home country was also hardly comparable as the population of the former was much bigger: In 1901, British India had almost 300 million inhabitants with an additional 3.5 million people living in Ceylon, whereas the population of the United Kingdom amounted to roughly 41 million.[59] The spread of a narcotic habit in

---

56 James H Mills, "Cocaine and the British Empire: The Drug and the Diplomats at the Hague Opium Conference, 1911–12," *The Journal of Imperial and Commonwealth History* vol. 42, no. 3 (2014), 418.

57 Compare HC Deb 3rd April 1883 col. 1344, where even Sir Joseph Pease, Quaker and president of the Society for the Suppression of the Opium Trade, called the Indians "a friendly, if somewhat barbaric, people." In 1908, the Secretary of State for India when asked about the "spread of the cocaine habit among all classes" in the country replied that "[t]he traffic in the drug ha[d] already been placed under restrictions in provinces where there was evidence of extensive and improper use," HC Deb 19th July 1908 col. 379.

58 In Chapter II, we established that 35–112 kg of cocaine were imported into British India annually between 1904 and 1908.

59 "Census of the British Empire. 1901. Report with Summary and detailed Tables for the several Colonies, &col., Area, Houses, and Population," (London: Wyman & Sons, 1906), xviii.

the colony thus was considered significantly worse and brought back memories from the spread of the opium habit in China.

The answer lies somewhere in between. The circumstances of coca and cocaine consumption in Britain elaborated so far indicate that it had not been considered a noteworthy problem for public health for quite some time. At the same time, the British attitude prevailed that the Indian people were more susceptible to develop a narcotic habit. This is reminiscent of the dealing with the opium and morphine habit some years prior: It was not considered a problem in the home country but significant enough in the colony to arrange a Royal Commission of Opium in the 1890s to investigate the matter. In conclusion, this points towards an explanation already given above. Rather than outsourcing a problem, Britain adopted stricter regulations in India out of fear for their moral progress as a seemingly less civilised population that required paternalistic guidance: The opium traffic, but also narcotic traffic in general, "debased the mind, degraded the character, and ruined the health. It was not only a stigma and a disgrace, but a real moral danger to the British Empire."[60]

Regardless of the motifs for stricter regulations in the colony, the members of the Cocaine Committee made an interesting suggestion concerning restrictions for coca products that did not occur in the home country. To them, their addictive potential seemed neglectable due to the low cocaine content, wherefore restrictions on specific products such as Hall's Coca Wine, Armbrecht's Coca Wine, Burrough & Wellcome's Voice Tabloids, and Tucker's Asthma Fluid should be loosened.[61] This distinction illustrated a more educated medical opinion on the topic that did not appear as relevant for England or other European countries that had become increasingly convinced of coca products after the 1860s. The committee's suggestion might have stemmed from the fact that coca products were never as popular in India since they did not have sufficient time to increase in popularity before cocaine entered their market.

Although some historians such as Alzada Comstock and C Knick Harvey have argued that Britain abandoned mercantilist practices in the mid-nineteenth century, they are still strongly reminiscent in coca and cocaine trade reg-

---

60 HC Deb 6th May 1908 col. 345. See also House of Commons, *Statement exhibiting the Moral and Material Progress and Condition of India during the Year 1874–75* (London: Eyre and Spottiswoode, 1876), 17, where it is stated that "It is not possible to stop the consumption [of narcotics, KE] altogether" as it would lead to illicit trade and consumption which was considered "conduci[ve] to demoralisation."

61 Cocaine Committee, "Opium, Morphia, and Cocaine," 8.

ulations in India in 1910.[62] The laws ruled that pharmacists and medical practitioners were only allowed to buy cocaine from European or Indian companies up to a quantity of one ounce and they also limited competition with products from the United States, for example, which were on the rise in the early twentieth century. In order to secure economic advantages in the coca trade, the state still played a significant role in directing economic activity and preventing foreign competition. Britain was well aware that the American cocaine industry posed a severe threat to British and European products.

As a result, they continued to exploit India in two ways after they had just settled the opium question: growing the raw product and selling it the manufactured product. Coca was cultivated on a small scale in several parts of the colony and the Indian government established factories in Bengal and Madras to produce cocaine.[63] This way, they reduced costs resulting from exporting the raw product and importing the purified product and ensured that the manufacturing process was confined to the British Empire. India was not only cocaine producer but also cocaine consumer which flushed money into British pockets. But in restricting imports from foreign companies, Britain's protectionist trade policy in India not only safeguarded British but also European cocaine industries but also played a significant role in their agreeance with Germany in the International Opium Conference 1912.

The mercantilist and protectionist practices of the British were further enhanced by confining the power to purchase cocaine only to those pharmacists and medical practitioners in India who practiced Western medicine. This also illustrated once again the cultural inconsideration inherent in cultural dissimilation that always accompanied the history of coca and cocaine in the British Empire. Whereas Western medicine was often associated with modernity and the progress of science, forbidding those who did not practice it to access cocaine products posed a devaluation of traditional or alternative treatment options and a disparagement of the Indian medicinal culture in general.

Even after the convention in Shanghai, Britain did not consider withdrawing from the narcotics trade or limiting their imports to Asia until at least May 1910. The recommendations issued by the commission were just that for the

---

62 Alzada Comstock, "British Economic Policy: I. Mercantilism," *Current History* 19, no. 109 (1950), 138; C Knick Harley, "Trade: Discovery, Mercantilism and Technology," in *The Cambridge Economic History of Modern Britain*, ed. Roderick Floud and Paul Johnson (Cambridge: Cambridge University Press, 2004), 176.

63 Government of India, Revenue Department, 31st October 1890, No. 857, 1, 3, 5.

British: recommendations. In accordance with the stalling tactic in the opium trade, Britain also tried to benefit from the cocaine revenue as long as possible. John Anderson wrote in a letter to the Earl of Crewe, dated 30th March 1910, that it was not even clear if Britain would participate in another conference concerning international drug control which indicated that Britain would not have taken action if it had been the only country to do so.[64] It required international pressure that Britain did not feel singled out to take action and accept pecuniary injuries in the narcotics trade which convinced them to participate in the convention at The Hague, as is explained further down.

According to the Consul General in Canton, British companies did not import cocaine into China or the Straits Settlement and blamed German company Merck for flooding the countries with their cocaine products after 1910.[65] This is ironic considering that Britain had forced opium on China for decades and ignored repeated requests to limit importation. It also was not true since Chinese Prince Ch'ing and the governments of Singapore and the Straits Settlement had repeatedly urged action to restrict cocaine imports but had not receive an answer for months. Another document on the "Production, Distribution, Sale, and Physiological Effects of Cocaine" also rejects that claim and stated that at the latest in 1903, Britain imported cocaine into India.[66] Superintendent F M Baddeley even went so far in accusing Britain of using bogus companies to import cocaine, mentioning deliveries labelled Lin Kee of London for which no company records could be found.[67]

When China issued an imperial edict to forbid cocaine imports for other than medicinal purposes, British diplomat Sir William Grenfell Max Müller in Peking finally wrote to Sir Earl Grey in February 1910 requesting to agree to that edict.[68] Surprisingly, Earl Grey initially saw no reason to do so or even to bring it up in the upcoming International Opium Conference, however, he also did not object to include it.[69] Germany equally published the translated version of the edict in July which must have meant that the only cocaine entering the country after 1910 must have been for its use in medicine.[70] There was cer-

64 John Anderson to the Earl of Crewe, 30th March 1910, letter, TNA.

65 Consul General to W G Max Müller, 11th July 1912, letter, TNA.

66 Dunstan, "Memorandum."

67 F M Baddeley to the Colonial Secretary, 1st June 1910, letter, TNA.

68 W G Max Müller to Earl Grey, 19th February 1910, letter, TNA.

69 W Langley to the Under Secretary of State, 13th May 1910, letter, TNA.

70 "Verordnung," newspaper cutting, 28th July 1910, TNA.

tainly a lot of cocaine smuggling in Asia in the first decade of the twentieth century but accepting the restrictions of Asian governments meant that foreign countries could not be blamed for promoting the habit on purpose. After having been the bogeyman in the opium trade in the nineteenth century, the focus shifted towards Germany as the culprit in the cocaine trade in the twentieth century.

5. The International Opium Convention at The Hague 1911/12

During the first years of the twentieth century, the United States grew increasingly concerned about the international drug trade as illegal narcotic consumption had turned out a severe threat to public health there. Other nations, such as China, who had similarly experienced the consequences of excessive narcotic consumption on their population, needed no convincing that there was urgent need for action. As a result, an International Opium Commission was convened by the United States in Shanghai in 1909 with the following other nations present: "Great Britain, Germany, France, Russia, Turkey, China, Japan, The Netherlands, Portugal, Siam, and Persia."[71] However, due to differing opinions on how to proceed with the global narcotic trade and the nature of the commission which did not hold the power to issue legal regulations, only recommendations were issued.

As this outcome was much to the dismay of prime movers of the commission, they urged for a successive meeting in form of a conference under leadership of the United States. As the Marquess of Crewe remarked: "That rapidity is really due to the fact that two years ago another Conference was held at Shanghai between representatives of the Powers, at which the whole question was fully discussed."[72] This time, though, the aim was to create an international drug treaty that all signing nations had to adhere to wherefore the Convention was set to convene in The Hague in December 1911. To expand the territorial validity of that first global drug treaty, not only the present nations – mostly those that had participated in the commission in Shanghai apart from Turkey

71 Paul S Reinsch, "Diplomatic Affairs and International Law, 1909," *The American Political Science Review* 4, no. 1 (1910), 51.

72 HL Deb 14th February 1912 col. 41.

who was substituted by Italy – were able to sign, but also "[a]ny Power not represented at the Conference."[73]

In the face of the International Opium Convention at The Hague, British politicians consulted medical professionals for their opinion concerning narcotic consumption in the British Empire.[74] As physicians prescribed those drugs and pharmacists dispensed them, they had a better understanding of the extent of narcotics consumption both in the home country and abroad to arrive at a well-developed answer to the question whether a spreading habit was reason for concerned. When it came to coca and cocaine they argued that the native habit of coca chewing was not comparable to the cocaine habit practiced by Europeans: "The danger of this practice is not comparable to that of the European habit of swallowing or injecting the alkaloid or its salts. It follows that whilst among the Indians over-indulgence is comparatively rare, among Europeans the cocaine habit is in the front rank of drug cravings."[75] Although contradictory to this statement, they recommended to include coca and issue the same restrictions as for cocaine. This is remarkable: Joint restrictions facilitated their enforcement but an even better motif was that the illegalisation of both substances instead of just one ensured that not only Britain but also no other state could engage in its trade.

Some historians such as William McAllister and Paul Gootenberg have argued that this motif was Britain's hidden agenda to get rid of competition in the narcotic trade, especially of Germany who became the centre of pharmaceutical research in Europe.[76] They claimed that Britain did not want to be the only country taking a significant loss due to the severe limitation of the opium trade

---

73 League of Nations, *International Opium Convention*, particularly invited were "all the Powers of Europe and America [...], that is to say: The Argentine Republic, Austria-Hungary, Belgium, Bolivia, Brazil, Bulgaria, Chile, Colombia, Costa Rica, the Republic of Cuba, Denmark, the Dominican Republic, the Republic of Ecuador, Greece, Guatemala, the Republic of Haiti, Honduras, Luxemburg, Mexico, Montenegro, Nicaragua, Norway, Panama, Paraguay, Peru, Romania, Salvador, Serbia, Spain, Sweden, Switzerland, Turkey, Uruguay, and the United States of Venezuela," 30.

74 HL Deb 14th July 1908 col. 569; Committee on Poisons, House of Commons, *Minutes of Evidence taken before the Departmental Committee appointed by the Lord President of the Council to consider Schedul A. to the Pharmacy Act, 1868, to report the Alterations therein which they deem expedient, and whether a third part should be added thereto; together with Appendices and Index to Evidence. Part II.* (London: Wyman & Sons Ltd, 1903), 24, 25, 158.

75 Dunstan, "Memorandum," 16th November 1909.

76 Mills, "Cocaine and the British Empire," 401, 402.

which would have left Germany with the upper hand. Consequently, Britain urged to include coca and cocaine in the draft which seemed to support their theory but another explanation seems more likely. This lay in Britain's position as a global power that had plenty of experience in the narcotic trade. As a world empire, Britain did not merely want to follow the suggestions of other countries concerning the global drug trade but to lead political action, since it was not yet ready to abandon its superiority: "Let Great Britain wait for no one but lead the way," as MP William Johnson declared.[77]

It is true – and this work has repeatedly addressed the issue – that Britain's dealing with narcotics was characterised by supremacist views and a strong interest to uphold the revenue drawn from them.[78] However, if commercial interests had still played such a significant role for the British in the 1909, it would have been smarter to only accept restrictions that would not endanger that goal. Like opium and morphine, Britain supported that coca and cocaine should solely be used for medicinal purposes which contradicts this theory. In addition, there was no evidence in the minutes of the conference where Britain hesitated to go forward with this decision. Quite on the contrary, as US delegates explained: "The British proposals in regard to morphine and cocaine were eminently sound, practical, and essential, and it became the duty of the International Opium Conference to provide against the abuse of morphine and cocaine similarly as regarded opium."[79] Consequently, "After the British Government made it a sine qua non that their participation in the International Opium Conference would depend upon [...] [this addition, KE] all the interested Governments willingly assented to this proposal [...]."[80]

77 HC Deb 6th May 1908, col. 345.

78 As PM William Gladstone said in 1840: "I have already stated, that although the Chinese were undoubtedly guilty of much absurd phraseology, of no little ostentatious pride, and of some excess, justice, in my opinion, is with them, and, that whilst they, the Pagans, and semi-civilized barbarians, have it, we, the enlightened and civilized Christians, are pursuing objects at variance both with justice, and with religion," HC Deb 8th April 1840 col. 819. This quote was re-iterated in future debates: 3rd August 1869 col. 1195, 4th June 1880 col. 1228, 3rd April 1883 col. 1337. Also compare PM Benjamin Disraeli in 1880: "The Indian revenue never can be solid and substantial so long as it is largely dependent on the opium revenue," HC Deb 4th June 1880 col. 1228.

79 Hamilton Weight, "Report from the Delegates of the United States to the Secretary of State," Department of State, 15th May 1912, accessed 18th June 2025. https://history.state.gov/historicaldocuments/frus1912/d307.

80 Weight, "Report from the Delegates," 15th May 1912.

Moreover, Britain sought private conversations with Germany during breaks to make sure they were on the same page, and MPs later highlighted the importance of the British-German friendship.[81] Historian James Mills equally argued that "nowhere in it [the conference, KE] [was] there a hint that the UK's representatives sought to provoke the Germans" but that "the opposite seems to have been the case."[82] As he further explained, "the British had not simply passed up an opportunity to secure commercial advantages. They had dismissed a proposal by the Germans that could have offered an easy way out of agreements [...]."[83] If anything, it seemed as if the British were more determined to reach agreements on international control of narcotics than Germany.

When concerned with their supremacist views, however, Mills claimed that Britain's change of heart might have stemmed from a feeling of guilt towards the Chinese after decade-long wrongdoing in the opium trade.[84] This explanation is unlikely. Despite repeated debates in both Houses of Parliament on the opium question, most MPs remained in favour of the opium trade even until the beginning of the twentieth century. Notions on the suffering of Asians due to opium usually came from politicians with a strong religious background who also favoured teetotalism. MPs such as Colonel Charles Yate, for example, claimed that "there [wa]s no more harm in such use of it [opium, KE] than there is in the afternoon cup of tea" which aligned with some "Indian and Colonial officials" who were similarly apathic towards anti-opium efforts, as MP Ernest Bennett argued.[85] In contrast to that, Theodore Taylor urged his fellow MPs not only to "help China to get rid of the opium in her own country" but to "banish it for ever from the whole territory of the British Empire."[86] This imbalance of opinions in British politics was never resolved in the long nineteenth century despite several efforts to change their minds, for example with the creation of a Royal Commission on Opium. It seems as if the feeling of supremacy was still deeply ingrained in most British minds so that feelings of guilt towards lesser developed countries on their behalf seemed utopian. This circumstance did not only play an important role in the proceeding of restrictions on narcotics but

81 HL Deb 14th February 1912, col. 40.

82 Mills, "Cocaine and the British Empire," 404.

83 Ibid., 408.

84 Mills, "Cocaine and the British Empire," 410, 413.

85 HC Deb 6th May 1908 col. 370; HC Deb 26th July 1911 col. 1717.

86 HC Deb 6th May 1908 col. 352.

also in the foreign narcotic trade. Even more so, since Britain was convinced that these countries bore part of the blame since they did not enforce the laws more strictly.

Britain's change of mind in the narcotic policy was caused by international pressure that resulted in a bandwagon effect. Rather than initiating stricter regulations of narcotics, Britain decided to concur with the overwhelming majority of nations in the International Opium Conference 1912 in order not to lose its image as a colonial benefactor. For more than a century, it had been the European power known for its reckless approach in forcing opium onto China but this attitude was not appropriate anymore after sociocultural and medicinal changes in the early 1900s. The professional world and the public alike were well aware that narcotics could cause addiction and it was the governments' task to limit access to such drugs to preserve and protect public health.

This development became very clear when the US showed that its primary interest was not the augmentation of narcotic revenue but the public health of its people which stood in sharp contrast to Britain's attitudes that prevailed until the conference. The rise of illicit narcotic trade and consumption, as well as the spread of addiction in the US was reason enough for the country to take action. Although public health had also improved in Britain over the decades, parliamentary debates showed that the country still struggled to put public health before British economic interests. The US was one step ahead of Britain since they realised the growing threat of addiction to public health and several states issued laws against the importation and sales of narcotics as early as 1877.[87] To insist on its attitude to uphold the narcotic trade as it was would have been detrimental for Britain's economy and political relations which left them with only one option: to concur.

Moreover, in painting cocaine with the same brush as opium and morphine regarding international drug control, Britain saw a chance to chapter out those people who posed a threat to its polished self-image: little-educated and morally inferior drug addicts. However, the actual consumers were not those that Britain suspected: Cocaine consumers were not previous opium consumers. As explained in Chapters III and IV, accessibility and affordability of cocaine in the Victorian Era was limited, so the consumer circle of this

87 William L White, "Race and Class in Early Anti-drug Legislation in the United States," accessed 18th June 2025, https://www.chestnut.org/Resources/74897b96-2909-4f2a-b927-809fb765fd06/Race-and-Class-in-Early-Anti-drug-Legislation-in-the-United-States.pdf.

specific narcotic shifted considerably from that of opium consumers. Opium was for the masses, cocaine was not. But British supremacy cared little for this distinction since the image of the socially and morally despicable drug addict still prevailed. An addict was an addict, no matter the drug consumed. But after investigating further and revealing that it was in fact upper class citizens who developed a dependency on cocaine after medical treatment or who used it as a recreational drug, this posed a threat to their moral reputation. For the past decades of the nineteenth century, they had witnessed the spread of the opium habit among the working class which they associated with a weakness of character and immorality and to be put into the same category as opium addicts was to be avoided at all costs.[88] Therefore, it was easier to hush the circumstances of cocaine consumption and paint it with the same brush as opium and morphine. It was a welcome diversion of attention away from the problems of seemingly well-educated and morally impeccable citizens to those who had already been used to public degradation. Narcotics consumption in the different social classes therefore played a much bigger role in Britain's change of mind than previously anticipated.

88 Compare MP Sir Joseph Pease: "[...] this drug [opium, KE] is demoralizing [...]," HC Deb 3rd April 1883 col.1343 and Theodore Taylor: "[...] [T]here is no European gentleman or lady who would like to be called an opium smoker. It would be an insult to anyone to have such an epithet thrown at him," HC Deb 27th June 1912 col. 593.

Addendum: The Career of Vegetable Narcotics

Looking back at the different chapters of this book it becomes evident that coca underwent five stages which I term the *Career of Vegetable Narcotics*: a botanical, economic, pharmaceutical, sociocultural, and political stage. It was necessary for botanists to examine the plant to determine its value for humanity and whether this value was sufficient to establish trade with its countries of origin. In order to conduct further experiments that could conclude in patent medicine, merchants had to be aware of proper storage and transportation to facilitate overseas trade. Successively, trade routes and means had to be determined, as well as taxation and additional regulations concerning the product. Only upon the arrival of bigger amounts of coca could pharmaceutical chemists develop medicine from the drug and collaborate with physicians who would then test it on their patients. As the new drug was introduced into the British market, society responded to it in specific ways that contributed to the creation of a coca culture that was entirely different from the native coca culture in South America. Only a few decades after its introduction, risks and dangers of the purified version of coca became known which called for political action and formed the last stage of coca's career in nineteenth-century Britain.

At this point, I would like to draw attention to one of the first cycles for psychotropic substances that was developed by neurologist Max Seige (1880–1969). In 1912, he developed the eponymous Seige Cycle and divided it into three stages.[1] In the first stage, high expectations accompany the excitement over the discovery of a new psychotropic substance which leads to its widespread use. In stage two, the novelty drug experiences increased criticism, particularly if expectations were not met, before in stage three, restrictions limit the drug's sales and consumption. This last stage then leads

1 Seige, "Klinische Erfahrungen mit Neuronal," 1828–30.

to a partial or complete disappearance from the market, but it is possible that the cycle surrounding this substance begins anew at some point in the future.

There are a few similarities and several differences in Seige's and my model that concern the existence of an actual cycle versus a progression, and the scope. First and foremost, my model of *Career of Vegetable Narcotics* assumes that the career of a narcotic progresses over time and changes throughout that process while Seige described a closed and reoccurring cycle of those psychotropic substances. In a way, one could argue that the rediscovery of coca in the nineteenth century confirms his claim that the cycle can start again from the beginning but this is where we disagree. Coca as a narcotic was rediscovered after some 300 years but when it appeared on the British market it experienced some sort of transformation through a changed mode of consumption and extended possibilities for its application. This was facilitated by medicinal developments such as the extraction of its alkaloid but also by the introduction of syringes, wherefore it makes more sense to speak of a progression rather than a cycle that has no clear beginning and no definite end.

Seige's model also does not leave the possibility that a narcotic can produce another, possibly riskier, narcotic. In his eyes, this new narcotic would require its own cycle. But the purification is part of a raw material's history, they are closely linked to each other. Without coca there would not be cocaine and without opium there would not be morphine, or even synthesised narcotics such as heroin. Purified products cannot account for rediscovery or reoccurrence since they have not previously existed. This does not mean that they do not face similar expectations, criticism, and restrictions, but there is a prelude to them that guided those and therefore a model to describe a narcotic's career in history must encompass its botanical origins. This guidance is facilitated by a continuous comparison between the raw material, i.e., the plant, and the purified substances to draw conclusions about their usefulness, applications, and risks to public health.

Consequently, the career of a narcotic clearly has a beginning and I do not believe that it is ever going back there to undergo the three phases anew, as Seige explained for his cycle. Coca's rediscovery sparked expectations but as I already pointed out above, these expectations were not the same the Spaniards had when they first encountered the coca culture in South America in the sixteenth century. British society did not expect coca to alleviate altitude sickness or suppress hunger but it was expected to become a popular reviving tonic – both in a medicinal and recreational aspect. Similarly, coca did not face criticism because it was considered a native vice, but because its alkaloid caused addiction in (British) people. Last but not least, restrictions on coca did not stem from its consumption being 'heathenous' and a *bête noire* in the eyes of the Anglican Church, as it was for the Catholic Church some centuries prior, but because from the dangers of its alkaloid. Seige did not argue that the expectations, criticism, and restrictions necessarily need to be the same when the cycle reoccurs, so it seems as if his model is temporarily and spatially independent but this is where our opinions diverge.

In excluding cultural circumstances, Seige failed to realise that his cycle cannot be applied to any narcotic at any time in any country or society and neither does it reoccur in various places at various times. For millennia, there were no disappointed expectations or rising criticism among coca-consuming populations in South America and until this day, some countries have not even issued any restrictions on coca. It was the encounter of different cultures that led to those changes because an indigenous vice suddenly had to be turned into a legitimate indulgence for Western populations overseas. This obvious imbalance of the social backgrounds of its consumers was another reason that influenced coca's career. Throughout history it was not the only narcotic that experienced this fate. Opium consumption was similarly widespread in the ancient Mediterranean world without any negative implications until it met with central European opposition after millennia-old use. It was this clash of cultures that facilitated a negotiation of narcotic consumption in the 'new' consumer countries. It was a clash of seemingly barbaric and civilized practices that fostered rethinking of the superior society. This rethinking was necessary because the medicinal value of those narcotics was simply too high to be abandoned.

These circumstances led to my claim that a narcotic career is more of a continuous process due to continuous influences and circumstances that accompany the (re)discovery, introduction, and career of a narcotic on the market. The few comparisons between coca and opium – and we might as well include other narcotics like Cannabis – show that their careers have rather progressed in stages. Both South American and Mediterranean populations first explored the botany of the drugs and their effects on the human body before they were cultivated and commodified. Coca lingered much longer in the botanical stage than opium because it was a daily necessity and not primarily a remedy. In Egypt, for example, opium quickly became a valuable commodity due to its proximity to other foreign countries that facilitated trade. This circumstance also enabled the transition to the pharmaceutical stage in which opium was marketed as medicine. Although opium had been banned in Europe in the Middle Ages, upon its rediscovery the British could pick up where antiquity left off: expanding the pharmaceutical market of opium and creating an opium culture. Coca, on the other hand, remained in a local economic stage before it expanded to a broader economic stage, i.e., overseas trade, and entered the pharmaceutical stage after the European re-encounter with the drug. Successively, it was influenced by sociocultural circumstances and eventually, both drugs and their purified products faced political restrictions. At this point, I would like to mention that some South American countries where coca has always been completely legal have not yet made it to this 'final stage' and maybe never will. However, it becomes clear that a model in which the career of a narcotic is continuously progressing seems much more reasonable as it can be transferred to different times and places.

Critics could argue that the last stage of my model, the political one, is superfluous because some narcotics such as coca might never reach it and they might also question whether this stage can even count as development. I claim that progress can also take on the form of restrictions, particularly if they are for the benefit of humanity, and that they do not contradict each other. The primary reason for British politics to limit the sales and consumption of narcotics was to prevent the spread of addiction and decrease mortality rates from poisoning, although fear of moral deterioration certainly played a role as well. Governments need to understand their responsibility for the public health of their citizens, so by issuing laws concerning narcotics, they set boundaries between beneficial and harmful. This does not go to say that all narcotic laws fulfil this premise, as we have witnessed with cannabis during the last few years, but they can at least serve as a guideline. If we take the Victorian Era as an example, many people were unaware of addiction or potential risks of overdoses, so the Pharmacy and Poisons Acts sought to implement preventative measures. Political regulations can also change over time as they adapt to new scientific findings. If we understand the last stage of my career model as being ever evolving due to its adaptability to changing circumstances, it is easy to see why it needs to remain in place.

Whereas Seige's cycle also included political aspects and therefore emphasised their importance in the career of a narcotic, it lacked the botanical, economic, and sociocultural stages in my model. This does not seem reasonable since it is essential to look at a substance's botanical origins and economic circumstances because they lay at the root of it all, quite literally. If there was no soil to grow and cultivate the new 'vegetable drug' coca, chances for mass production were limited. Similarly, if there was soil but it lay outside the imperial realm, trade relations had to be established and terms of trade defined in the first place to enable mass production. Without the botany and economy, which created the basis for the introduction of a novelty drug on the British market, a Seige cycle cannot even evolve. Consequently, Seige thought his cycle too narrow-minded in merely focusing on a new narcotic that was already widely available.

The question of availability then brings me to the sociocultural circumstances he had left out in his model. In assuming the three As – availability, accessibility, and affordability – Seige painted all narcotics with the same brush. While all three have been fulfilled for opium, this was not true for coca and certainly not for cocaine for at least three decades. In previous chapters, I have pointed out that the consumption of those drugs, especially of cocaine, was mostly confined to the well-to-do which indicates that the Seige cycle portrayed the career of a narcotic as one for the upper classes rather than for the population as a whole. If we turn this around and try to fit opium – *the* Victorian drug – into his cycle, this can be confirmed. Britain was opium-sodden and particularly fond of 'their' narcotic since it was a panacea for plenty of ailments and grown in the British Empire. As a result, expectations soon reached a plateau and criticism was at a minimum despite a high number of opium poisonings. There were certainly critical voices, such as that of the Anti-Opium Society, but they did not come from the vast working class and neither was it them that fostered political regulations on the drug. Criticism and limitations proceeded from religious activists and from those that had influence, i.e., the upper classes, wherefore the Seige cycle does not depict the career of a narcotic in society as a whole.

The only part where our models overlap is that the career of a narcotic or psychotropic substance cannot be explained without the medicinal value for the people and their reaction to it. As research into novelty drugs and medicinal developments progressed, knowledge about coca increased significantly, gave scientists insights into the potency of its alkaloids, and opened up possible avenues for their application. Seige was right that this sparked expectations that have exceeded the limitations of coca and cocaine's use and therefore caused disappointment. This disappointment was certainly part of the criticism but most of the criticism that emerged was due to the dangers that became known later on. Nineteenth-century medicine still relied on trial and error on humans for the most part, so it was hardly surprising that ignorance of correct doses of cocaine caused poisoning or even death. Eventually, as Seige rightfully explained, this led to restrictions of their consumption and sales although the effects of coca and cocaine differed significantly.

Exactly one hundred years after Seige, another explanation for the evolution of narcotics on the market was proposed by social historian Hans Derks. Coining it the 'Opium Problem' and focusing on this narcotic alone, he explained that there existed six different questions that were dealt with over time: a producer/production, a quality, a consumer, a sociocultural, a moral, and a legal opium question. Derks claimed that "[t]his original six-fold Opium Problem developed in history in the sense that new elements were added, but nothing of the original complexity was lost. After the second half of the nineteenth-century especially, the medical and pharmaceutical elements were added in both Europe and Asia."[2] In its complexity, this concept is closer to my *Career of Vegetable Narcotics* than Seige's model and it also accounts for economic and "medical and pharmaceutical elements" in a similar way.

However, Derks' concept cannot be universally applied for several reasons. Firstly, in focusing on opium alone, he limited the scope of this concept while at the same time expanding it by examining the role of Britain, the Netherlands, France, Japan, and the United States.[3] He argued that their inclusion was crucial since they "can provide us with the necessary details, definitions of an Opium Question and comparisons."[4] However, the amount of countries needed to explain the trajectory of opium from the seventeenth to the twentieth century neglects that each and every one of these countries faced different circumstances. These accompanied the trade of the drug, its introduction into the local market, the manufacturing and marketing of these products, the reception by respective populations, and ultimate restrictions. His view is therefore limited to an examination of how these actors contributed to the so-called 'opium problem' rather than how the career of this drug evolved in one specific country.

Secondly, as a six-fold problem that it was from the very beginning according to Derks – albeit a few elements being added over the course of time – this neither constitutes a cycle, as Seige suggested, nor progress, as proposed in my model. This makes his history of opium rather inflexible to changes and influences and creates a problem in itself. It also creates the impression that all six

2 Derks, *History of the Opium Problem*, 713.

3 Ibid., v-vii.

4 Ibid., 32.

aspects were relevant at the same time, when in fact, they were emphasised independently. This was equally true for the history of opium as for the history of coca investigated on the previous pages. Derks' legal opium question, for example, might have been raised early on within a small frame during the seventeenth century but it massively gained in importance during the global drug conferences in the early twentieth century. Besides, his producer/production opium question was certainly answered by then.

Last but not least, it remains unclear whether any of the six aspects he outlined disappear or increase in importance in due course. In highlighting new elements that can be added, Derks implied that they were rather attachments to the six-fold self-contained 'problem.' Nevertheless, in merely adding a medical and/or pharmaceutical element to this initial 'problem,' for example, this severely undermines the role of medicinal developments and the role of the pharmaceutical industry for a drug on a market, as I have shown. In this regard, Derks also claimed that "the western pharmaceutical industry and science had replaced the traditional herbal knowledge and experience."[5] This is not true. The western pharmaceutical industry has not replaced but *transformed* traditional herbal knowledge. Opium and coca have not disappeared from the market and at least the latter has not been replaced. Their modes of consumption changed and later their derivate morphine and alkaloid cocaine, respectively, increased in popularity. Moreover, traditional herbal knowledge of those vegetable narcotics is still very common in their originating countries and has resisted western pharmaceutical influences.

The predetermined stages of my model then raise questions as to its compatibility with the rather flexible network theory and its interdependencies. What seems like a contradiction at first works well if we understand the development of the coca network as a template for the model. The expansion of the coca network happened naturally since other professions had to enter the network to foster the career of the drug any further when existing competencies did not suffice. Botanists did not have the knowledge about trade, so they needed wholesalers and merchants to acquire coca overseas and transport it back to Britain. Neither botanists nor traders knew enough about creating medicine out of raw material, so chemists and pharmacists became additional actors in the network. Successively, neither of these professions had the authority to limit the trade, sales, or consumption of coca and cocaine for the sake of public health wherefore politicians were the last profession to enter the

5 Ibid., 722.

coca network. In a way, this evolution can be separated into stages that were accompanied by network mechanisms such as reciprocity and transitivity to illustrate how the foci in the career of a narcotic shifted over time. Both the evolution of the coca network and my model for the *Career of Vegetable Narcotics* do not interpret these stages as rigid and self-contained – the transitions are fluid and interdependencies between the different actors persist. The stages merely emphasise specific professions that were responsible for the continuous promotion of coca and cocaine. This progression led to an expansion of the network rather than causing a loss of relationships even when some actors passed away and were substituted by descendants, friends, or colleagues.

I repeatedly compared coca and opium to explain my model of the *Career of Vegetable Narcotics* – since they both produced significantly stronger purified products and confirmed my findings – but it is still necessary to conduct further research into the careers of other narcotics in the nineteenth century to support or contradict my model. It is desirable to investigate if part of my model can be applied to synthetic narcotics as well, for example to heroin that was created in the twentieth century. Furthermore, the timeframe of the two narcotics mentioned above on the British market differed greatly from around 50 years for coca to over 100 years for opium which raises questions as to the overlapping or interfering of the stages with each other during a longer time span that could be answered in future studies of the subject. In addition, it could be helpful to find out more about the circumstances and contributing factors that led to an extension or shortening of the stages for other drugs.

Conclusion

Almost all people have a desire to consume drugs to facilitate life, especially when they alleviate pain in one way or another. People also strive to discover more and better drugs that are safer, more affordable, and easier to administer. However, the drugs people choose for that purpose and the amount they are taking is up to each individual. On a macro level, this is influenced by culture, on a meso level by society, and on a micro level by an individual's upbringing as well as their physical and mental disposition. As a result, drugs are constantly influenced by cultural, social, economic, and political circumstances and are an essential part of human life. History has shown that we cannot paint every narcotic with the same brush which requires an evidence-based analysis of published and unpublished sources rather than a synthesis or re-evaluation of historiography and literature. This is especially true for coca whose history has recently focused on its career as an illegal drug in the globalised world. Starting out as an exotic narcotic in South America, coca had been used for millennia by the native population before it entered the British market, just like opium about a century prior, but they were then forbidden at the same time. To examine coca as a commodity that arrived in Europe with a lot of potential but received comparatively little attention in nineteenth-century Britain, this made for an intriguing analysis that was at the heart of this book.

The history of coca dates back millennia when it was considered the sacred leaf of the Inca and primarily used in religious ceremonies. Over time, it became a valuable drug for the whole population due to its nutritious properties and it relieving altitude sickness in the Andes. In the early nineteenth century, coca was rediscovered by European botanists after it had been a lucrative commodity for the Spanish during the Iberian conquest of South America in the sixteenth century. Recognising its value for human health from millennia-long use of Andean populations, explorers such as von Tschudi, von Martius, Weddell, or Markham contemplated its value for European populations.

Shortly after its rediscovery, Britain started to evaluate the possibility of cultivating coca in the vast British Empire to be independent of the trade with Peru and Bolivia. It had to overcome the challenge that coca required specific geographical characteristics to yield sufficient crops. To that aim, a network evolved from the Royal Botanical Gardens at Kew who not only supplied botanists in British colonies with coca seeds and specimens, but also with knowledge about proper cultivation thereof. Within only two decades, this network expanded to include chemists, wholesalers, and traders who examined the leaves' potential for the pharmaceutical market and potential trade routes. From the 1860s to the 1880s, this network originating at Kew flourished through a connection of various actors in the British Empire who worked diligently on coca becoming a British commodity. However, as economic and pharmaceutical aspects became more important, the role of the network gradually diminished.

Cultivation efforts in the imperial realm initially turned out unsuccessful for the most part wherefore pre-existing trading relations between Britain and South America, and between Britain and Asian countries could have facilitated entering the coca trade. Nevertheless, while the opium trade with Asia commenced in the eighteenth century and rapidly gained momentum in the nineteenth century with a peak at the *fin de siècle*, trade with coca only started out in the mid-nineteenth century and would not by a long stretch reach the same extent. This is especially remarkable since Britain engaged in competition with Germany and France who had entered the coca trade with Peru some years prior. Bills of Entry show that the main port of entry for coca in Britain was Liverpool, with lesser amounts arriving at the port in London, and that a few deliveries were in transit to Hamburg, Germany. Coca was imported into Britain after the 1870s and reached its peak in the 1890s when deliveries occurred on a more regular basis, about bi-monthly. Still, the amount imported remained insignificant in comparison to that imported into Germany or France around the same time. Even the purification of the drug did not change the comparatively low numbers of imported coca and cocaine. Despite these circumstances, Britain later took advantage of their trade routes to British India in exporting coca and cocaine to the colony. Trade was an essential part of the career cycle of a drug in the home country, since without continuous supply, consumption declined and national revenue decreased.

The contrast in the coca trade between Britain and mainland Europe became even more evident with the discovery of cocaine that was highly dependent on the coca supply. Challenges concerning the transportation of coca leaves across the Atlantic Ocean, such as loss of potency due to improper storage and lengthy journeys, had delayed research on coca in Europe although Italian scientist Paolo Mantegazza had already conducted research on coca in Peru in the mid-nineteenth century. When the first significant amount of coca arrived overseas in the late 1850s, German scientist Albert Niemann extracted its alkaloid cocaine shortly after and noted its anaesthetic properties. In Britain, Sir Robert Christison also experimented with the leaves and found a crystallisable amount but until the 1870s, he did not have sufficient leaves to pursue this further to confirm Niemann's findings.

The breakthrough only happened with the discovery of cocaine as a local anaesthetic by Carl Koller in 1884 when its hypodermic application acted as a juggernaut for the prominence of cocaine. As a consequence, the pharmaceutical industry acted quickly on that development in creating a range of coca and cocaine products for the wider public. Coca wine, coca and cocaine lozenges and tablets were among the most popular products as they were more affordable than pure cocaine and syringes to administer it subcutaneously. In Britain, Allen & Hanburys took the leading role but over the years advertising in the media greatly contributed to the sales of products of other companies as well. However, the discovery of cocaine increased not only the potency but also the dangers of accidental overdoses which the medical profession increasingly warned about. Contrasting coca, cocaine, and their impact on the drugs' role in British society showed that it was not the purification alone that made coca an exceptional narcotic but rather a changed mode of consumption.

This changed mode of consumption then demonstrates that coca underwent cultural dissimilation. South American people resisted supremacist influences in continuing their millennia-old practices of chewing coca leaves and drinking coca tea against altitude sickness and as a digestive, but Britain decided to rather dissolve coca leaves in alcohol and use it as a reviving tonic. Later on, when cocaine entered the market, it was swallowed as tablets, drunken in a solution, or administered hypodermically which was far from how the coca leaf was originally consumed. As a result, the coca leaf became a cultural marker for Andean populations and has remained a valuable commodity in its traditional use in South America until this day.

Although the amount and kind of drugs consumed in Britain varied greatly throughout the social classes, public media gave important insights into the wider trends over the course of the long nineteenth century as it influenced public opinion and vice versa. Newspaper articles provided the public with information on products available on the market, where to get them, and informed about the desired effects of the new medicine. Occasionally, they also warned of negative side effects such as physical and mental deterioration which might lead to addiction. Contrasting the reception of both drugs in British and German media illustrated different attitudes towards the drugs, since in Germany they were received more euphorically than in Britain. It showed that the respective populations were part of bigger medicinal and social movements that occurred during the last decades of the Victorian Era, especially with Germany becoming the centre for cocaine production and leaving Britain behind.

The influence of Victorian fiction for the career of coca in Britain could also not be neglected as it raised awareness for negative consequences of overindulgence in narcotics. Fictional characters such as Sherlock Holmes, Dorian Grey, and Dr Jekyll illustrated that initially medicinally induced cocaine (and also opium) consumption could lead to a habit that turned into a vice and eventually, became a disease called addiction. Besides from physical deterioration, the authors also wanted their readers to realise how this behaviour deteriorated morality and created social misfits. This attitude was also taken up by the temperance movement which promoted total abstinence of any drug that could impact one's health and therefore urged for the inclusion of coca and cocaine in political regulations later on. Contributing to that were not only the fictional portrayals of criminal addicts but realistic crimes for which doctors were sued, such as alleged cocaine poisoning and cases in which cocaine was used to intentionally taking one's own life or that of somebody else.

The continuously improving knowledge about the effects of narcotics on the human body, the evolution of the concept of addiction, and the concern on behalf of other Western nation about their detrimental consequences for public health then acted as a juggernaut for legal restrictions on both coca and cocaine at the beginning of the twentieth century. Initially, Britain only adopted stricter measures in India where cocaine smuggling and a so-called cocaine habit were on the rise. Due to prevailing imperialistic attitudes, the motherland felt the need to restrict the consumption of coca and cocaine in its colony in order not to threaten moral progress of a population they had considered uneducated and uncivilised for quite some time. Unsurprisingly, this was the primary concern in both Houses of Parliament when cocaine consumption, among other narcotics was debated. The realisation that narcotic consumption could be a threat to public health in general, regardless of class and ethnicity, stemmed from increasing concerns on behalf of other Western countries such as the United States. Eventually, several countries convened in international conferences in 1909 and 1911/12 to discuss global restrictions on narcotics. These led to both coca and cocaine facing the same fate as opium and morphine when they were both declared illegal for other than medicinal purposes. The brief outline of the proceedings at the Commission on Narcotic Drugs at the United Nations Conference in Vienna 2023 demonstrated that the missing distinction between coca and cocaine has still not been resolved today after more than 110 years.

As an addendum, I offered a concept for the career of so-called 'vegetable' drugs in the nineteenth century based on the research conducted. I claim that those drugs undergo five phases that evolve from one another and whose transition is fluid: a botanical, economic, pharmaceutical, sociocultural, and political phase. Its flexibility lies in its ability to emphasise different aspects at different times that ensures that all components are addressed based on the priorities in each phase. This does not go to say that one phase was more important than the others – all phases are essential for the career of a vegetable narcotic. In the case of coca, cultivation opportunities had to be ensured before establishing trade routes and connections that would then facilitate scientific research and the development of pharmaceutical products. Consumer behaviour, their habits, and attitudes towards coca products would then determine its success or failure on the market, particularly under the influence of advertisement. British politicians concurred with international opinion that coca needed to be painted with the same brush as cocaine and other narcotics such as opium and morphine. This opinion has not changed until this day, although scientific research revealed that coca leaves do not contain a significant portion of the narcotic agent that react with the human body in a way that would cause serious health problems or addiction.

A comparison with other concepts developed by Seige and Derks then demonstrated that the *Career of Vegetable Narcotics* can serve as a template for the dealing with other vegetable narcotics that have just been introduced into the market or are yet waiting to be (re-) discovered. My concept differs from Seige's cycle, in which three successive phases repeat each other with the discovery of more potent derivates or alkaloid of a specific drug, as the careers of narcotics are *not* considered cyclical. Seige also skipped the botanical and economic prelude of the career of narcotics, though they are essential for the success or failure of a new drug on the market. Drawing on more research on narcotics in history – given the one hundred years gap – Derks developed a more comprehensive concept that understands narcotics as a multidimensional 'problem' that has added elements over the course of centuries.

However, he included several countries that contributed to this so-called 'opium problem' which blurred the lines of the distinct histories of opium in those countries. Although in here, I also just focus on the history of one particular drug, namely coca, my model suggests that it is applicable to other vegetable narcotics as well. As such, it can provide a valuable contribution to the history of narcotics in general.

This work joins the ranks of other histories on singular narcotics, such as Berridge's and Edwards' *Opium and the People* or Gootenberg's *Andean Cocaine* while it refrained from writing a singular cultural or economic history. Instead, understanding the history of coca as an entangled history expands the methodological canon as it encompasses various aspects that have previously been neglected or only dealt with on the periphery. To that end, it utilised published and unpublished sources such as Bills of Entry, parliamentary papers, and consular reports that have been overlooked by other researchers but provide a valuable contribution. At the same time, it did not disregard the comparison to other drugs like opium and to other countries like Germany and France for better contextualisation, although these comparisons did not reach the same extent as in Courtwright's *Forces of Habit*, for example.

Rather than looking at how cocaine became illegalised in a top-down approach, I conducted a causal investigation to distinguish between coca and cocaine and to trace the career of the former in nineteenth-century Britain from the bottom up. As a result, this approach turned out more adaptive as assumptions and hypotheses could be adjusted with the gathering of additional evidence. Gootenberg, for example, claimed that Britain just arrived too late on the colonial scene to become a major player in the global coca and cocaine trade, when in fact, the circumstances were way more complex.[1] In addition, keeping this flexibility helped to understand the dynamic processes that influenced coca's career in Britain, particularly revealing the influence of the network surrounding Kew that might otherwise have been overlooked. Whereas this bottom-up approach accounted for the complexities of the history of coca, it did not lose sight of the illegalisation that accompanied the history of coca later on.

Critics could argue that the entangled history of coca can merely scratch on the surface due to its nature of examining a variety of aspects. This study has shown that the contrary is the case. The shift in foci over time emphasised crucial influences for coca's career in Britain, identified key problems in the

1 Paul Gootenberg mentioned this in personal communication.

respective fields, and explained how they were addressed. Rather than forming a collection of different histories, this facilitated a better focus of depth.

It might also occur to some historians that the United States' role in the career of coca and cocaine was underrated here although it was the juggernaut for global restrictions for the two drugs in the twentieth century. At the same time, it can be objected why references to Germany, France, and Asia were necessary. Whereas the first claim is not wrong, the history of coca and cocaine in the US differed greatly from that in Britain and Europe which requires its own research. References to other countries were indispensable for this analysis as they highlighted similarities and differences in the perception of coca, the coca trade, coca consumption, medical developments, and political regulations.

Future research wants to dive deeper into the history of coca in nineteenth century France and Germany where the drug has sparked much enthusiasm and where crucial medicinal research on the drug took place. In doing so, this can reveal where the *Career of Vegetable Narcotics* I developed is applicable to those countries as well and if the career of coca faced the same influential circumstances there. Moreover, applying my concept to the history of other narcotics can prove or refute its validity and reliability. Further research might also give a better insight into the roles of class and gender in the history of coca and explain how it fits in into the evolution of the concept of addiction in the Victorian Era.

Most desirable is, though, that future research on coca focuses more on the raw material rather than the purified cocaine. The effects of the coca trade on Andean culture, society, economy, and politics from the Iberian conquest until today provide a plethora of starting points for more extensive research that can contribute to a re-evaluation of the negative perception of the coca leaf in the twenty-first century.

Essay: A Study of Coca Historiography

The following essay gives readers interested in the history of narcotics an overview of literature in the field that has concentrated on coca and/or cocaine in a variety of contexts. Given that opium has had a considerably earlier and longer history in Britain, this bias in literature is not surprising but neglects the fact that there were other drugs who equally deserve researching, preferably in a comparative approach with a global outlook. This does not only concern the big three – alcohol, tobacco, and caffeine – but also the little three – Opium, Cannabis, and Coca, as coined by David T Courtwright.[1] It is coca in particular that has received little attention due to a deeper interest into its more potent alkaloid cocaine and the accompanying drug crisis in the twentieth century.[2] However, it is the sociocultural and medicinal roots of this modern cocaine history that require a closer look by nineteenth-century historians. A recent request of South American countries to exclude coca from the narcotics schedule at the United Nations Conference in Vienna mid-March 2023 sparked renewed interest in the motifs for its prohibition roughly 111 years ago at the International Opium Commission at The Hague 1912 and the history leading up to it.[3]

The rediscovery of coca as a valuable drug in the early nineteenth century was accompanied by a fascination of the 'exotic.' Scientists such as Angelo Mariani highlighted coca's marvellous properties as medicine which successfully

1 Courtwright, *Forces of Habit*.

2 For a brief overview of the Global War on Drugs in the twentieth century, see Maria Mcfarland Sánchez-Moreno, "Winding Down the War on Drugs: Reevaluating Global Drug Policy," *Harvard International Review* 36, no. 4 (2015): 35–39.

3 For more information about the most recent conference see "Sixty-sixth session," United Nations Office on Drugs and Crime, accessed 18th June 2025, https://www.unodc.org/unodc/en/commissions/CND/session/66_Session_2023/66CND_Main.html.

promoted the sale of his coca products.[4] It discussed botanical prerequisites for coca cultivation, a variety of applications as a medicine, and several pharmaceutical products that could be obtained by consumers. Due to the nature of the book, which can be counted as advertisement for Mariani's products, it is marked by an absence of negative connotations regarding the dangers of coca consumption, such as side effects or overdoses in conjunction with alcohol. This idealisation therefore refrained from a critical approach towards the drug while neglecting cultural and economic circumstances.

William Golden Mortimer was then the first historian who processed the interpretation of the exotic plant in greater detail.[5] In no less than sixteen chapters, Mortimer delineated the history of coca in a comprehensive approach from the Incas to his contemporaries, highlighting geographical and botanical aspects of the plant, as well as its religious and medicinal applications. As a doctor, he argued for the benefit of coca's actions on the human body and provided examples for its use in food and medicine. Mortimer's book was an attempt to idealise the drug at a time when the production of its alkaloid cocaine and negative side effects thereof overshadowed the previously proclaimed beneficial properties of coca leaf. As such, it argued in the same line as Mariani – except from pushing the sales of specific pharmaceutical products – while also neglecting the economic and social downsides of the introduction of coca into European societies. Both seemed to want to liberate coca from its stigma that evolved with the spread of cocaine but at the same time involuntarily or purposefully disregarded legal consequences of this development.

Despite or because of debates surrounding narcotics in general in the first decades of the twentieth century with the International Opium Commission in Shanghai in 1909 and the International Opium Convention in The Hague in 1911, it is hardly surprising that this time is marked by an absence of interpretations of the history of coca alone. A shift towards a disparaging interpretation of coca and cocaine, among opium, morphine, and cannabis, was then characteristic of the early twentieth century.[6] In his book, Collins claimed that these drugs posed the biggest threat to public health as they caused addiction and led

4 Angelo Mariani, *Coca and its Therapeutic Applications* (New York: J. N. Naros, 1896).

5 William Golden Mortimer, *History of Coca – "The Divine Plant" of the Incas* (J. H. Vail: New York, 1901).

6 Cornelius Francis Collins, *The drug evil and the drug law* (New York: M.B. Brown, 1918).

to moral deterioration. Whereas he focused on the spread of illicit consumption in the United States and consequential legal restrictions, Collins' work illustrated that the world grew increasingly concerned about narcotics and realised that politics needed to take action to avoid a public health crisis.

The decades between the First World War and the late-twentieth century were marked by an absence of research on the history of narcotics. This could have been due to global conflicts at the time which included two World Wars, challenges during the Reconstruction Era, and the Cold War when research topics shifted towards other fields of interest. Renewed interest in drugs for recreational use arose after the 1970s when several historians continued the tradition of writing a social or sociocultural history of coca and published this as part of a broader discussion of drugs.[7] With Brian Inglis leading the way, he claimed spirits, opium, hemp, heroin, and cannabis as the most influential drugs in world history while coca and cocaine only received little attention on a few pages.[8] Similarly, Terry M Parssinen dealt with the role of cocaine in the history of drugs only in passing and completely neglected the history of coca.[9] This is even more surprising since he focused his research on British society between 1820 and 1930 when both coca and cocaine were novel narcotics on the market and would have deserved a closer look. However, they explain how sociocultural factors shaped the careers of drugs in history and how they evolved from medicinal necessities to recreational substances.

An exception in the contemporary discussion of various psychoactive substances was Joseph Kennedy who concentrated on coca and cocaine alone.[10] Furnished with a plethora of prints, photos, drawings, and advertisements, he provided a more accessible and less exaggerated interpretation than Mortimer and shed light on the history of coca from the Inca in the first century AD to problems caused by cocaine in contemporary American society. Nevertheless, Kennedy took the same line as Mariani and Mortimer in idealising not only coca but also cocaine which he both considered 'safe' drugs in moderate use. He also disregarded the economic history of coca that played an important role

7 A much earlier attempt to compromise the history of certain narcotics in *The Seven Sisters of Sleep* by botanist Mortdecai Cooke was published in 1860 but it had not yet dealt with coca as one of the most prominent narcotics at the time. This is hardly surprising as coca products only entered the British market in successive years.

8 Inglis, *The Forbidden Game*.

9 Parssinen, *Secret Passions, Secret Remedies*.

10 Joseph Kennedy, *Coca Exotica: The Illustrated Story of Cocaine* (London: Associated University Presses, 1985).

for the availability of the drug in Europe in the nineteenth century and focused on political restrictions on both coca and cocaine in the United States. Still, Kennedy's collection of visual representations of the history of coca is beyond comparison.

Since the illicit global trade in narcotics occupied the minds of politicians and public health officials with the emergence of an opioid and cocaine crisis, especially in the United States in the 1990s and early 2000s, historians opened their research to more than a single narcotic. David T Courtwright, for example, named cocaine as one of the "little three" psychoactive substances next to opium and cannabis.[11] Although he focused on cultural aspects of a total of six psychoactive substances in world history, he also included economic and political dimensions evolving from their careers. Jordan Goodman, Andrew Sherratt, and Paul E Lovejoy similarly offered a comprehensive overview.[12] Expanding Courtwright's six psychoactive substance by yagé and kola nuts, the authors also approached the history of narcotics from a cultural perspective. Courtwright, Goodman, Sherratt, and Lovejoy all claimed that these substances have shaped not only local cultures but the global cultural landscape in creating habits that cause problems in public health. Consequently, their analysis adds to the interconnectedness of culture and drugs. Given the extent of the topic in both books, though, treatments of the economic and political circumstances of the history of coca are underexplored and fall under the general explanation of narcotics trade and restrictions.

However, the turn of the twentieth to the twenty-first century simultaneously experienced a shift towards the history of cocaine due to the drug's rise during globalisation. To this day, cocaine remains the mostly consumed illicit drug in Europe, right after Cannabis, and the amount of illegal seizures have increased annually.[13] Steven B Karch then traced back the history to the encounter of the Spanish conquistadores with coca and successively argued how the drug made it to Europe and became popular there.[14] Karch primarily fo-

11 Courtwright, *Forces of Habit*.

12 Jordan Goodman, Andrew Sherratt, and Paul E Lovejoy, *Consuming Habits: Global and Historical Perspectives on How Cultures Define Drugs: Drugs in History and Anthropology* (Florence: Taylor & Francis Group, 2007).

13 European Union Drugs Agency, "Understanding Europe's drug situation in 2024 – key developments (European Drug Report 2024)," accessed 18th June 2025, https://www.euda.europa.eu/publications/european-drug-report/2024/drug-situation-in-europe-up-to-2024_en.

14 Karch, *A Brief History of Cocaine*.

cused on medicinal and pharmaceutical consequences of the discovery of cocaine and corresponding legislative consequences. His history of cocaine then concluded with a focus on the United States and Japan with the rise of illegal cocaine trade in the twentieth century. In writing a history of cocaine rather than a history of coca, Karch followed a product-oriented approach that emphasised the alkaloid of coca instead of the leaf itself.

A more recent treatment of the history of cocaine can then be found in Paul Gootenberg's works which the author called "an antidote to these received and mainly superficial accounts of cocaine."[15] A prominent name among historians researching narcotics, Gootenberg sought a cliometric approach that emphasised economic and political aspects accompanying the history of cocaine.[16] Given the titles and content of his works, it becomes clear that Gootenberg understands coca and cocaine as two different drugs, arguing that the first is for local and the latter for global use.[17] Whereas his books demonstrate a profound knowledge of the history of cocaine along the South-American-North-American axis, the role of both coca and cocaine in European societies, particularly in England in the nineteenth century, was neglected.

When analysing the history of coca, and narcotics in general, it is essential to also look at the evolution of medicine and pharmacy as developments in the respective fields influenced the careers of those drugs. More specifically, the evolution of the concept of addiction deserves special attention as it reveals more about availability of the drugs on the market, their consumers, and consequential effects on legal restrictions. Louise Foxcroft thus attempted a textual approach to examine how addiction evolved as a concept.[18] She utilised fictional and non-fictional literature to explain addiction from a cultural and medical point of view but focused on opium as the primary narcotic causing this disease. However, fiction always tends to distort reality and conclusions as to the understanding of addiction must therefore be drawn with caution. A better explanation of addiction had already been published almost three

15 Paul Gootenberg, ed., *Cocaine: Global Histories* (London: Routledge, 1999); Gootenberg, *Andean Cocaine*.

16 Cliometrics is a methodology that evolved in the 1950s and 1960s that sought to apply "economic theory and quantitative methods to the study of economic history," Claude Diebolt and Michael Haupert, "Cliometrics: Past, Present, and Future," *Association Francaise de Cliométrie* Nr.4 (2021), https://hal.science/hal-03345558/document, 1.

17 Gootenberg, *Andean Cocaine*, 10.

18 Louise Foxcroft, *The Making of Addiction: The 'Use and Abuse' of Opium in Nineteenth-Century Britain* (Burlington: Ashgate Publishing Company, 2007).

decades prior by Virginia Berridge who covered a longer period of time and included more than just opium as a narcotic that caused addiction at that time.[19] Berridge delineated how the concept of addiction evolved in Britain from a medicinal point of view and claimed that the medical profession had to enter a partnership with the government to agree on a "moral-*cum*-medical" theory of addiction which resulted in a much more beneficial narcotic policy in Britain than in the United States, for example.[20] This article explains how developments in medicine, particularly regarding narcotics, informed political actions and how they were co-dependent.

In the last fifteen years, renewed interest arose in the long-forgotten value of coca leaves which the overwhelmingly overshadowing illicit trade in cocaine had blurred. Therefore, Irmgard Bauer argued from a medicinal perspective how coca back then as today has been used by Andean population to help with altitude sickness and digestive problems, thus posing a natural and affordable alternative to modern processed and costly medicine.[21] She rightfully claimed to "rehabilitate" coca, as it does not cause by far the addiction attributed to its alkaloid cocaine, and has proved itself as a valuable plant for millennia. Similarly, Victor B Stolberg described the use of coca and asserted its relevance for South American ethnic groups.[22] The same year, Philip Reiser published an article in which he traced the history of coca from its use in ancient rituals to the problems it caused in modern-day society.[23] All three authors share the opinion that coca leaves themselves are not the problem – it is what is done with

19 Virginia Berridge, "Morality and medical science: Concepts of narcotic addiction in Britain, 1820–1926," *Annals of Science*, Volume 36, Issue 1 (1979), 67–85.

20 Berridge, "Morality and medical science," 68; cursive in the original. The Harrison Act in the United States 1914 ruled that physicians were not allowed to treat addicts, thus contributing to an underground network. In Great Britain, however, there was no restriction regarding treatments but restrictions applied to who was allowed to dispense narcotics, in what amount, and to whom. As early as 1868, the Pharmacy Act ruled that dispensers needed to keep a register with this information which facilitated the enforcement of such restrictions. See Chapters III and V.

21 Irmgard Bauer, "Travel Medicine, Coca and Cocaine: Demystifying and Rehabilitating *Erythroxylum* – a Comprehensive Review," *Tropical Diseases, Travel Medicine and Vaccines* 5 (2019), 1–14.

22 Victor B Stolberg, "The Use of Coca: Prehistory, History, and Ethnography." *Journal of Ethnicity in Substance Abuse* 10, no. 2 (April 2011), 126–46.

23 Philip Reiser, "The Drug Industry in Peru: From Sacred Leaves to Political Curse." *KAS International Reports (Konrad Adenauer Stiftung)*, 8 (2011), 7–21.

them in illegal workshops and illegal overseas trade and consumption that has caused economic and political problems.

Whereas their research is much appreciated to set the record straight in making a distinction between legal coca leaves (at least in South America countries) and illegal cocaine, it did not deal with coca specifically in nineteenth-century Britain. This omission was partly rectified by Bettina Wahrig.[24] As a historian of pharmacy and science, Wahrig outlined the use of coca and later cocaine in the nineteenth century as medicine which initially provided a seemingly useful antidote to opium and morphine addiction.

The literature on coca and cocaine discussed here demonstrates that the history of those drugs has received interest in specific aspects. The cultural history of coca at the time of the Inca in South America is well-researched, covering its use in ancient rituals and the Spanish encounter with the drug, as well as coca's role as a cultural marker to this day. Researchers have also dealt with the significance of the discovery of cocaine in the nineteenth century and its implications for medicine and pharmacy both in Europe and the United States. In addition, several comparative studies situate cocaine among other psychoactive substances, thus contributing to patterns in the history of narcotics, finding differences and similarities, and enabling cross-disciplinary insights. Of particular interest has been cocaine as an illegal drug in and after the twentieth century, which compromised economic as well as political aspects, that have called for global restrictions to eliminate public health risks. As the United States took on a leading role in the fight of illicit cocaine trade early on, it has been the centre of attention for many modern researchers of narcotics.

In addition to the literature discussed in this essay, this work then traced the introduction of a commodity that previously served as a cultural marker for a native population onto the British market. Although not as widely used as opium (another narcotic) or tobacco (another drug made from leaves), it also explained rising consumerism that had since been disregarded in historiography. [25] It gave new insights into the interaction between consumer desires and

---

24 Bettina Wahrig, "'Fabelhafte Dinge': Arzneimittelnarrative zu Coca und Cocain im 19. Jahrhundert." *Berichte zur Wissenschaftsgeschichte* 32 (2009), 345–364.

25 As John Benson stated, "there [was] a desire, above all, for that which [was] new, modern, exciting and fashionable" to which Peter Stearns added that, starting in the late eighteenth century, many people "[...] shopped around for remedies, with more consumerist zeal, perhaps, than their descendants would display, confined as the latter were by a firmer commitment to scientific medicine," compare John Benson, *The Rise of Consumer Society in Britain, 1880–1980* (London, 1994), 4; Peter N. Stearns, "Stages of

the commercialisation of a 'vegetable drug' and enriched our understanding of how lesser-studied commodities shaped patterns of consumption in nineteenth-century Britain.

Researchers interested in the history of narcotics may now want to focus on origin stories of modern-day natural drugs which could be of value in the future and which might lead to more well-informed verdicts in drug policies worldwide. The field of medicine and pharmacy has experienced a giant leap during the past 150 years wherefore it comes as a surprise that the raw materials for many drugs are still painted with the same biased brush as their manufactured products. Cannabis, for example, has just stepped out of the shadow as a morally deteriorating recreational drug to become an addition to the medicinal palette of pain relief. With due diligence, historians can help that society and politics also realise this potential for coca after it has been vilified for at least the last century.

Consumerism: Recent Work on the Issues of Periodization," *The Journal of Modern History* 69, no. 1 (1997), 106, 107.

Bibliography

Published Sources

Books

General List of Drugs, Pharmaceuticals, and the "Allenburys" Specialties. London: Allen & Hanburys Ltd., 1908.

Reise der Oesterreichischen Fregatte Novara um die Erde, in den Jahren 1857, 1858, 1859 unter den Befehlen des Commodore B. von Wüllerstorf-Urbair. Beschreibender Theil. Dritter Band. Wien: Kaiserlich-Königliche Hof- und Staatsdruckerei, 1862.

Acosta, Joseph. *The Naturall and Morall Historie of the East and West Indies.* Translated by E. G. London: Printed by Val: Sims for Edward Blount and William Aspley, 1604.

Bidie, G. *Coca, its Source, Culture, Uses, &c.*, (with a Plate). Madras: Higginbotham & Co., 1885.

Blyth, Alexander. *Poisons: Their Effects and Detection. A Manual for the Use of Analytical Chemists and Experts.* London: Charles Griffin and Company, 1895.

Chemical Department. Processes (Book III). London: Burroughs, Wellcome & Co, 1908.

Chemical Department. Processes (Book IV). London: Burroughs, Wellcome & Co, 1908.

Cooke, Mortdecai. *The Seven Sisters of Sleep.* Rochester: Park Street Press, 1997.

De Cieza de León, Pedro. *Crónica del Perú: El Senorío de los Incas.* Edited by Franklin Pease G. Y. Caracas: Fundación Biblioteca Ayacucho, 2005.

De Quincey, Thomas. *Confessions of An English Opium-Eater. With "Levana", "The Rosicrucians And Freemasons", "Notes from The Pocket-Book of A Late Opium-Eater", Etc.* London: Walter Scott, 1886.

Doyle, Arthur Conan. *The Sign of Four.* London: Spencer Blackett, 1890.

Gaedcke, F. *Ueber das Erythroxylin,* dargestellt aus den Blättern des in Südamerika cultivirten Strauches Erythroxylon Coca Lam. Berlin: W. Moeser & Kühn, 1854.

Galvano, Antonie. *The Discoveries of the World from Their First Originall Unto the Yeere of Our Lord 1555.* Translated by Richard Hakluyt. London: Impensis G. Bishop, 1601.

Gorges, Ferdinando. *America Painted to Life. The True History of The Spaniards Proceedings in the Conquests of the Indians, and of their Civil Wars among themselves, from Columbus his first Discovery, to these Later Times.* London: Printed for Nath. Brook at the Angel in Cornhil, 1659.

Griffins, Arthur. *Mysteries of Police and Crime. A General Survey of Wrongdoing and its Pursuit.* Volume II. London: Cassell and Company Ltd, 1899.

Hooker, W. J. *Companion to the Botanical Magazine; Being a Journal, Containing such Interesting Botanical Information, as does not Come Within the Prescribed Limits of the Magazine; With Occasional Figures.* London: Botanical Magazine Warehouse, Essex, 1835.

Julian, Don Antonio. *La Perla de la America, Provincia de Santa Maria, Reconocida, Observada, y Expuesta en Discursos Historicos.* Madrid: Printed for Don Antonio de Sancha,1787.

Lamarck, M. le Chevalier de. *Encyclopèdie Méthodique. Botanique.* Tome Second. Paris: Panckoucke, 1786.

Lindley, John. *Natural System of Botany; or, a Systematic View of the Organisation, Natural Affinities, and Geographical Distribution, of the whole Vegetable Kingdom; together with the Uses of the most Important Species in Medicine, the Arts, and Rural or Domestic Economy.* London: Longman, Rees, Orme, Brown, Green, and Longman, 1836.

Mantegazza, Paolo. *Quadri della natura umana. Feste ed ebbrezze.* Volume II. Milano: Giuseppe Bernardoni, 1871.

Mariani, Angelo. *Coca and its Therapeutic Application.* New York: J. N. Naros, 1896.

Markham, Clements. *Travels in Peru and India.* London: John Murray, 1862.

Meyen, Franz J. F. *Outlines of the geography of plants: with particular enquiries concerning the native country, the culture, and the uses of the principal cultivated plants on which the prosperity of nations is based.* London: Printed for the Ray Society, 1846.

Mulhall, Michael G. *The Dictionary of Statistics.* London: George Routledge and Sons, Ltd., 1899.

Niemann, Albert. Über eine neue organische Base in den Cocablättern. Göttingen: E A Huth, 1860.

Poeppig, Eduard. *Reise in Chile, Peru und auf dem Amazonenstrome, Während der Jahre 1827–1832*. Leipzig: Friedrich Fleischer, 1836.

Pomet, Pierre. *A Compleat History of Druggs*, Written in French by Monsieur Pomet, Chief Druggist to the present French King, to which is added what is further observable on the same Subject, from Mess. Lemery, and Tournefort, Divided into Three Classes, Vegetable, Animal and Mineral; With Their Use in Physick, Chymistry, Pharmacy, and Several Other Arts. London: Printed for R. Bonwicke, William Freeman, Timothy Goodwin et al., 1712.

Reid, Mayne. *The forest exiles, or, The perils of a Peruvian family amid the wilds of the Amazon*. Boston: Ticknor and Fields, 1858.

Simmel, Georg. *Soziologie. Untersuchungen über die Formen der Vergesellschaftung*. Leipzig: Duncker und Humblot, 1908.

Stevenson, R.L. *The Strange Case of Dr Jekyll and Mr Hyde*. London: Longmans, Greens and Co. 1886.

Thackeray, William Makepeace. *The History of Pendennis*. London: Smith, Elder & Co, 1887.

Von Briba, Ernst Freiherr. *Die Narkotischen Genußmittel und der Mensch*. Nürnberg: Wilhelm Schmid, 1855.

Von Martius, C. F. P., ed. *Reise in Brasilien auf Befehl Sr. Majestät Maximilian Joseph I. Königs von Baiern in den Jahren 1817 bis 1820 gemacht von weiland Dr. John. Bapt. Von Spix und Dr. Carl Friedr. Phil. von Martius*, Dritter und letzter Theil. München: Friedr. Fleischer, 1831.

Von Tschudi, J. J. *Travels in Peru, During the Years 1838–1842, on the Coast, in the Sierra, across the Cordilleras and the Andes, into the Primeval Forests*. Translated by Thomasina Ross. London: David Bogue, 1847.

Weddell, H. A. *Voyage Dans le Nord de la Bolivie et dans les Parties Voisines du Perou ou Visite au District Aurifère de Tipuani*. Paris: P. Bertrand, 1853.

Wilde, O. *The Picture of Dorian Gray*. London: Harper Collins, 2010.

Zárate, Augustin de, and Martin Nucio. *Historia del des cubrimiento y conquista del Peru, con las cosas naturales que senaladamente alli se hallan, y los sucessos que ha audio*. Casa de Martin Nucio, 1555.

Government Papers

"Census of the British Empire. 1901. Report with Summary and detailed Tables for the several Colonies, &c., Area, Houses, and Population." London: Wyman & Sons, 1906.

A Collection of the Public General Statutes Passed in the Thirty-First and Thirty-Second Years of the Reign of Her Majesty Queen Victoria: Being the Third Session of the Nineteenth Parliament of the United Kingdom of Great Britain and Ireland. London: Eyre & Spottiswoode, 1868.

Bueno, Emilio Arce de la Torre. "Discurso del Presidente Ejecutivo de Devida, en la Sesion plenaria CND." United Nations 66th session of the Commission on Narcotic Drugs, Vienna. March 2023. Accessed 18th June 2025, https://www.unodc.org/documents/commissions/CND/CND_Sessions/CND_66/Item_3_-_Peru.pdf.

Choquehuanca, David. "Descolonizar la Hoja de Coca en el Tiempo de Pachakuti." United Nations 66th session of the Commission on Narcotic Drugs, Vienna. March 2023. Accessed 18th June 2025. https://www.unodc.org/documents/commissions/CND/CND_Sessions/CND_66/Item_3_-_Bolivia.pdf.

Choquehuanca, David. "Palabras Inaugurales." United Nations 68th session of the Commission on Narcotic Drugs, Vienna. March 2025. Accessed 20th August 2025. https://estatements.unmeetings.org/estatements/31.0365/20250310100000000/KntrDKxQ/DMloUx-kUlW_vna_es.pdf.

Cocaine Committee. "Opium, Morphia, and Cocaine." 29th August 1912. TNA.

Committee on Poisons. House of Commons. *Minutes of Evidence taken before the Departmental Committee appointed by the Lord President of the Council to consider Schedul A. to the Pharmacy Act, 1868, to report the Alterations therein which they deem expedient, and whether a third part should be added thereto; together with Appendices and Index to Evidence. Part II.* London: Wyman & Sons Ltd, 1903.

Coroner's Committee. House of Commons. *Report of Inquiry Into the Question of Deaths Resulting from the Administration of Anaesthetics.* London: Eyre and Spottiswoode, 1910.

Customs Bill of Entry Liverpool. 25th August 1855 – 10th July 1899. London: British Library.

Customs Bill of Entry London. 1st June 1880 – 20th December 1900. London: British Library.

Government of Bolivia. "World Health Organization Critical Review of the Coca Leaf Supporting Dossier." Accessed 20th August 2025. https://hojadecoca.cancilleria.gob.bo/wp-content/uploads/2023/09/Coca-Review-Dossier-Annex-English-revised-VP-240523.pdf.

Government of India. "Extract from the Abstract of Proceedings of Council, dated 8th November 1905. The United Provinces Excise Law Amendment Bill, 1905."

Government of India. Legislative Department. "Annexure to Bill to amend the Excise Act, 1896."
Government of India. Revenue Department. "Accompaniments to Government Resolution." 3rd July 1908, No. 6666.
Government of India. Revenue Department. 31st October 1890, No. 857.
Government of Madras. Revenue Department. 27th March 1885, No. 385.
HC Deb 3rd April 1883, vol. 277, col. 1333–1363.
HC Deb 4th April 1843, vol. 68, col. 361–469.
HC Deb 6th June 1907, vol. 175, col. 900–914.
HC Deb 6th May 1908, vol. 188, col. 339–380.
HC Deb 8th April 1840, vol. 53, col. 748–837.
HC Deb 10th May 1870, vol. 201, col. 460–534.
HC Deb 13th May 1901, vol. 93, col. 1456–1457.
HC Deb 19th July 1906, vol. 161, col. 352–532.
HC Deb 21st July 1909, vol. 8, col. 497–594.
HC Deb 24th May 1895, vol. 34, col. 278–324.
HC Deb 26th July 1911, vol. 28, col. 1645–1786.
HC Deb 27th June 1912, vol. 40, col. 463–638.
HC Deb 29th April 1881, vol. 260, col. 1451–1514.
HC Deb 30th June 1893, vol. 14, col. 591–634.
HL Deb 1st August 1839, vo. 49, col. 1052–1074.
HL Deb 2nd February 1843, vol. 66, col. 29–30.
HL Deb 3rd August 1894, vol. 28, col. 1–5.
HL Deb 4th June 1857, vol. 145, col. 1091–1101.
HL Deb 4th June 1858, vol. 150, col. 1507–1516.
HL Deb 5th April 1906, vol. 155, col. 617–671.
HL Deb 5th March 1857, vol. 144, col. 1881–1892.
HL Deb 7th April 1859, vol. 153, col. 1505.
HL Deb 7th February 1895, vol. 30, col. 177.
HL Deb 9th March 1857, vol. 144, col. 2026–2050.
HL Deb 9th March 1869, vol. 194, col. 944.
HL Deb 9th May 1879, vol. 246, col. 1–8.
HL Deb 12th March 1857, vol. 144, col. 2196–2209.
HL Deb 12th May 1840, vol. 54, col. 1–48.
HL Deb 14th February 1912, vol. 11, col. 1–47.
HL Deb 14th July 1908, vol. 192, col. 537–580.
HL Deb 14th May 1857, vol. 145, col. 249–257.
HL Deb 15th June 1840, vol. 54, col. 1166.

HL Deb 15th June 1868, vol. 192, col. 1556.
HL Deb 15th July 1912, vol. 12, col. 486.
HL Deb 15th May 1879, vol. 246, col. 390.
HL Deb 17th May 1847, vol. 92, col. 917.
HL Deb 19th February 1861, vol. 161, col. 548–570.
HL Deb 19th February 1895, vol. 30, col. 1061–1066.
HL Deb 19th March 1858, vol. 149, col. 409–417.
HL Deb 19th March 1885, vol. 295, col. 1665–1678.
HL Deb 20th August, vol. 147, col. 1884–1887.
HL Deb 21st December, vol. 198, col. 2345–246.
HL Deb 21st May 1840, vol. 54, col. 460–486.
HL Deb 22nd June 1857, vol. 146, col. 106–136.
HL Deb 22nd May 1906, vol. 157, col. 1073–1107.
HL Deb 23rd August 1907, vol. 181, col. 1368–1372.
HL Deb 23rd July 1878, vol. 242, col. 1–38.
HL Deb 24th August 1857, vol. 147, col. 2003–2068.
HL Deb 24th August 1893, vol. 16, col. 930–932.
HL Deb 26th February 1857, vol. 144, col. 1319–1383.
HL Deb 29th June 1894, vol. 26, col. 532.

House of Commons. *Consumption of Opium in India*. London: Eyre and Spottiswoode, 1892.

House of Commons. *Diplomatic and Consular Reports on Trade and Finance. China. Report for the Year 1894 on the Foreign Trade of China*. London: Harrison and Sons, 1895.

House of Commons. *Diplomatic and Consular Reports on Trade and Finance. Peru. Report for the Year 1886 on the Trade of Mollendo*. London: Harrison and Sons, 1887.

House of Commons. *Diplomatic and Consular Reports on Trade and Finance. South America. Report for the Year 1887 on the Trade of Mollendo (Peru)*. London: Harrison and Sons, 1888.

House of Commons. *Diplomatic and Consular Reports on Trade and Finance. Colombia. Report on the Agricultural Condition of Colombia*. London: Harrison and Sons, 1888.

House of Commons. *Diplomatic and Consular Reports on Trade and Finance. Peru. Report for the Year 1888 on the Trade of Mollendo*. London: Harrison and Sons, 1889.

House of Commons. *Diplomatic and Consular Reports on Trade and Finance. Peru. Report for the Year 1890 on the Trade of Callao*. London: Harrison and Sons, 1891.

House of Commons. *Diplomatic and Consular Reports on Trade and Finance. France. Report for the Year 1890 on the Trade of the District of the Consulate General of Havre*. London: Harrison & Sons, 1891.

House of Commons. *Diplomatic and Consular Reports on Trade and Finance. Germany. Report for the Year 1886 on the Trade and Agriculture of Wurtemberg*. London: Harrison & Sons, 1887.

House of Commons. *Diplomatic and Consular Reports on Trade and Finance. Germany. Report for the Year 1889 on the Trade of the Consular District of Frankfort-on-Maine.* London: Harrison & Sons, 1890.

House of Commons. *Diplomatic and Consular Reports on Trade and Finance. Germany. Report for the Year 1890 on the Trade of the District of the Consulate-General at Frankfort.* London: Harrison & Sons, 1891.

House of Commons. *Diplomatic and Consular Reports on Trade and Finance. Germany. Report for the Year 1892 on the Trade, &c., of the Grand Duchy of Baden*. London: Harrison & Sons, 1893.

House of Commons. *Diplomatic and Consular Reports on Trade and Finance. Germany. Report for the Year 1895 on the Trade of Mannheim*. London: Harrison and Sons, 1896.

House of Commons. *Diplomatic and Consular Reports on Trade and Finance. Germany. Report for the Year 1907 on the Trade of the Consular District of Berlin*. London: Harrison and Sons, 1908.

House of Commons. *Diplomatic and Consular Reports on Trade and Finance. Peru. General Report for the Year 1896 on Peru*. London: Harrison and Sons, 1897.

House of Commons. *Diplomatic and Consular Reports on Trade and Finance. Bolivia. Report for the Year 1895 on the Trade, &c., of Bolivia*. London: Harrison and Sons, 1897.

House of Commons. *Diplomatic and Consular Reports on Trade and Finance. Colombia. Report for the Year 1896 on the Trade of Panama*. London: Harrison and Sons, 1897.

House of Commons. *Diplomatic and Consular Reports. Chile. Report for the Year 1901 on the Trade of Chile. (Supplementary.)*. London: Harrison and Sons, 1902.

House of Commons. *Diplomatic and Consular Reports. Peru. Report for the Year 1897 on the Trade of Callao*. London: Harrison and Sons, 1898.

House of Commons. *Diplomatic and Consular Reports. Peru. Report for the Year 1897 on the Trade and Finances of Peru*. London: Harrison and Sons, 1898.

House of Commons. *Diplomatic and Consular Reports. Peru. Report for the Year 1898 on the Trade and Finances of Peru*. London: Harrison and Sons, 1899.

House of Commons. *Diplomatic and Consular Reports. Peru. Report for the Year 1902 on the Trade of Peru*. London: Harrison and Sons, 1903.

House of Commons. *Diplomatic and Consular Reports. Peru. Report for the Year 1901 on the Trade and General Condition of Peru*. London: Harrison and Sons, 1902.

House of Commons. *Diplomatic and Consular Reports. Peru. Report for the Year 1905 on the Trade and General Condition of Peru*. London: Harrison and Sons, 1906.

House of Commons. *Diplomatic and Consular Reports. Peru. Report for the Year 1907 on the Trade and Commerce of Peru*. London: Harrison and Sons, 1908.

House of Commons. *East India (Consumption of Ganja)*. London: Eyre and Spottiswoode, 1893.

House of Commons. *East India (Trade). Review of the Trade of India in 1909–10*. London: Wyman & Sons, 1911.

House of Commons. *Report on the Indian Excise Committee 1905–06*. London: Darling & Sons, 1907.

House of Commons. *Report, Supplementary Report, and Minority Report of the Departmental Committee appointed by the Lord President of the Council to consider Schedule A. to the Pharmacy Act, 1868, to report the alterations therein which they deem expedient, and whether a Third Part should be added thereto, with a copy of the Minutes appointing the Committee, and a List of Witnesses examined. Pt. I (Pharmacy and Poisons: Sale of Poisons)*, by Herbert Eustace Maxwell, 6th Baron Monreith. London: Wyman & Sons, 1903.

House of Commons. *Statement exhibiting the Moral and Material Progress and Condition of India during the Year 1870–71*. London: Eyre and Spottiswoode, 1872.

House of Commons. *Statement exhibiting the Moral and Material Progress and Condition of India during the Year 1874–75*. London: Eyre and Spottiswoode, 1876.

House of Commons. *Statement exhibiting the Moral and Material Progress and Condition of India during the Year 1890–91*. London: Eyre and Spottiswoode, 1892.

House of Commons. *Statement exhibiting the Moral and Material Progress and Condition of India during the Year 1900–01*. London: Eyre and Spottiswoode, 1902.

House of Commons. *Statement exhibiting the Moral and Material Progress and Condition of India during the Year 1902–03*. London: Eyre and Spottiswoode, 1904.

House of Commons. *Supplement to the Thirty-Sixth Annual Report of the General Board of Commissioners in Lunacy for Scotland*. Edinburgh: Neill & Co., 1895.

House of Commons. *Tables Relating to the Trade of British India with British Possessions and Foreign Countries 1900–01 to 1904–05*. London: Wyman and Sons, 1906.

House of Commons. *Tables Relating to the Trade of British India with British Possessions and Foreign Countries 1901–02 to 1905–06*. London: Wyman and Sons, 1907.

House of Commons. *Tables Relating to the Trade of British India with British Possessions and Foreign Countries 1904–5 to 1908–9*. London: Eyre and Spottiswoode, 1910.

League of Nations. *International Opium Convention Signed at the Hague, January 23rd, 1912*. The Hague, 3rd April 1923. https://treaties.un.org/doc/Treaties/1922/01/19220123%2006-31%20AM/Ch_VI_2p.pdf.

Report of the Indian Excise Committee, 1905–06. London: Darling & Son, 1907.

Review of the Trade of India in 1909–10. London: Wyman & Sons, 1911.

Sarabia, Laura. "Intervención Debate General." United Nations 68th session of the Commission on Narcotic Drugs, Vienna. March 2025. Accessed 20th August 2025. https://estatements.unmeetings.org/estatements/31.0365/20250310100000000/KntrDKxQ/PIVEb-KEr_vna_es.pdf.

Savastano, S. E. Laura Gabriela Gil. "Debate General." United Nations 66th session of the Commission on Narcotic Drugs, Vienna. March 2023. Accessed 18th June 2025, https://www.unodc.org/documents/commissions/CND/CND_Sessions/CND_66/Item_3_-_Colombia.pdf.

The Monopolies Commission. House of Commons. *Report on the Supply of Cigarettes and Tobacco and of Cigarette and Tobacco Machinery*. London: Her Majesty's Stationary Office, 1961.

US Congress. *Congressional Record*. 30th Congress, 1st Session, 1848. Chapter 70: 237–239. Accessed 18th June 2025. https://maint.loc.gov/law/help/statutes-at-large/30th-congress/session-1/c30s1ch70.pdf.

Weight, Hamilton. "Report from the Delegates of the United States to the Secretary of State." Department of State, 15th May 1912. Accessed 18th June 2025. https://history.state.gov/historicaldocuments/frus1912/d307.

Articles

"(Ein neues Mittel gegen die Seekrankheit.)." *Hannoverscher Kurier*, 18th November 1885.

"(Zur Warnung)." *Hannoverscher Kurier*, 3rd December 1885.

"-." *Dortmunder Zeitung*, 6th December 1886.

"-." *Hallesches Tageblatt*, 15th February 1885.

"-." *Hannoverscher Kurier*, 11th April 1885.

"-." *Schwäbischer Merkur*, 20th November 1884.

""Coca Leaf."." *The Academy*, 11th October 1879.
"A Chymist and Druggist: The Sale of Poisons." *The Times*, 11th October 1856.
"A Costly Stimulus." *Once a Week*, 1st April 1876.
"A New Stimulant." *The London Review and Weekly Journal of Politics, Literature, Art, and Society* 3, no. 63 (14th September 1861): 329.
"A Pharmaceutical Chymist: Chymists and Druggists." *The Times*, 17th September 1856.
"Accident to the Prince of Wales. Injured While Out Shooting." *The Guardian*, 13th December 1895.
"Adulteration of Food, Drinks, and Drugs." *The Times*, 26th July 1855.
"Amerika. (Peru.)." *Karlsruher Zeitung*, 4th January 1826.
"Armbrecht Coca Wine." *The Times*, 24th February 1896.
"Aromatischen Coca-Liqueur." *Düsseldorfer Volksblatt*, 24th April 1877.
"Arzneikunde." *Dresdner Journal*, 15th May 1891.
"Asthma und Catarrhe der Luftwege." *Hannoverscher Kurier*, 25th November 1878.
"Außerordentlich weit hat man es jetzt in der Anwendung schmerzstillender Mittel gebracht..." *Chemnitzer Anzeiger und Stadtbote*, 14th March 1885.
"British Medical Association." *The Times*, 13th August 1886.
"Charge of Manslaughter by the Careless Administration of Laudanum." *The Morning Chronicle*, 13th April 1858.
"Chlorhydrate of Cocaine as an Anaesthetic." *Manchester Times*, 6th December 1884.
"Coca Praeparate." *Bonner Zeitung*, 8th November 1875.
"Coca." *The Planter's Gazette* (2nd March 1885): 203–204.
"Coca." *Chambers's Journal of Popular Literature, Science and Arts* no. 646 (13th May 1876): 318–9.
"Coca-Pillen I, II & III." *Echo der Gegenwart*, 14th April 1872.
"Cocain." *Hallesches Tageblatt*, 19th December 1885.
"Cocaine for Teeth-Pulling. A Druggist's Remorse." *The Guardian*, 23rd January 1908.
"Cocaine." *The Glasgow Herald*, 26th December 1884.
"Cocaine." *Chambers's Journal of Popular Literature, Science and Arts* 3, no. 114 (6th March 1886): 145–7.
"Cocaine as a Local Anaesthetic." *British Medical Journal* (6th December 1884): 1161–1162.
"Cocainismus." *Dresdner Nachrichten*, 27th February 1889.
"Coca-Präparate." *Karlsruher Zeitung*, 6th April 1873.

"Coca Wine and its Salts." *British Medical Journal* (6th February 1897): 353.
"Cocoa." *Journal of the Society of Arts*, 4th September 1868.
"Cucaine and its salts." *British Medical Journal* (13th December 1884): 1201–1.
"Das mörderische Cocain." *Bielefelder General-Anzeiger*, 16th January 1903.
"Das neue Heft der Annales du Commerce extérieur..." *Schwäbischer Merkur*, 3rd November 1866.
"Death from Cocaine." *The Morning Post*, 2nd July 1895.
"Death of a Clergyman from Cocaine Poisoning." *The Guardian*, 7th August, 1897.
"Der Cocainismus." *Kölnische Zeitung*, 29th August 1889.
"Der Fluch der Betäubungsmittel." *Hannoverscher Kurier*, 11th July 1886.
"Die erstaunlichsten Heilwirkungen..." *Kölnische Zeitung*, 23rd March 1876.
"Die Gefährlichkeit mancher modernen Heilmittel." *Berliner Börsen-Zeitung*, 20th August 1889.
"Die Herstellung des Cocains..." *Hallesches Tageblatt*, 29th December 1885.
"Die Reihe der anesthetischen (betäubenden) Mittel..." *Echo der Gegenwart*, 30th March 1862.
"Die wunderbaren Nähr- u. Heilkräfte..." *Rhein- und Ruhrzeitung*, 30th September 1875.
"Dr Charles Fauvel." *British Medical Journal*, Vol. 1 (11th January 1896): 118.
"Dr. medic. Samson's Coca-Pillen." *Echo der Gegenwart*, 13th March 1867.
"Drunkenness, Morphine, Opium & Cocaine Habits." *The Daily News*, 28th March 1893.
"Editorial." *Pharmaceutical Journal* 17 (1857/8).
"Ein neues Opiat." *Echo der Gegenwart*, 26th September 1861.
"Ein wunderbares Kräftigungsmittel." *Leipziger Tageblatt und Anzeiger*, 3rd October 1874.
"Eine lebhafte Conjunctur war für Cocain..." *Leipziger Tageblatt und Anzeiger*, 24th April 1885.
"Eine wunderbare Pflanze." *Dresdner Nachrichten*, 15th November 1866.
"Endlich legte D. Marquart ein Kästchen mit Cocablättern vor..." *Kölnische Zeitung*, 15th October 1861.
"Erfolge der Fahrt der "Novara."." *Bonner Zeitung*, 4th May 1860.
"Erkenntnisse eines Cocainisten." *General-Anzeiger für Dortmund und die Provinz Westfalen*, 19th December 1896.
"Fraud. Important Notice. Vin Mariani-Coca Wine." *The Era*, 5th May 1883.
"Free Test." *Longman's Magazine* (April 1897): 29.
"Great Britain and the Opium Traffic." *The Times*, 22nd September 1910.

"Hall's Wine (Hall's Coca Wine). A Marvelous Restorative." *The Guardian*, 6th April 1899.

"Hall's Wine (Hall's Coca Wine). A Marvelous Restorative." *The Guardian*, 20th April 1899.

"High Court of Justice. King's Bench Division. The Sale of an Asthma Remedy." *The Times*, 16th January 1908.

"Hydrochlorate of Cocaine, the new local Anaesthetic." *British Medical Journal* (29th November 1884): 1081.

"Im Bannes des Cocain." *General-Anzeiger der Stadt Mannheim und Umgebung*, 31st January 1908.

"In der Cocainnarkose." *Berliner Volksblatt*, 24th August 1888.

"Inquest. Cocaine for Tooth Extraction." *The Times*, 23rd January 1908.

"International Congress of Legal Medicine." *The Times*, 24th August 1889.

"King's Bench Division. Taylor and Wife v. The London Hygienic Institute. Alleged Negligent Administration of an Anaesthetic." *The Times*, 3rd November 1908.

"Kunst, Wissenschaft und Leben." *Kölnische Zeitung*, 13th September 1889.

"Literary and Other Notes." *The Guardian*, 6th December 1884.

"Locales. Die Gefährlichkeit mancher modernen Heilmittel..." *Berliner Börsen-Zeitung* (20th August 1889.

"Lungenleiden, Schwächezustände." *Kölnische Zeitung*, 2nd January 1870.

"Miszellen. Briefboten in Peru." *Bonner Zeitung*, 22nd March 1826.

"Mr. Gladstone's Eyesight. A Successful Operation." *The Guardian*, 23rd May 1894.

"Naturwissenschaftliche Volksbücher. VII. Die Chemie des täglichen Lebens." *Aachener Zeitung*, 20th April 1855.

"Neue americanische Medicamente des Special-Arztes Dr. Sampson aus New York." *Kölnische Zeitung*, 5th June 1866.

"Niederrheinische Gesellschaft für Natur- und Heilkunde zu Bonn." *Kölnische Zeitung*, 23rd March 1860.

"Nur Prof. Dr. Sampson's Coca Präparate..." *Echo der Gegenwart*, 17th September 1876.

"On the Sale of Poisons." *Pharmaceutical Journal* 4 (1844/5).

"Opium – Opium-Eaters – The Opium-Trade with China." *The Saturday Magazine* (November 1839).

"Oxford Circuit." *The Times*, 11th July 1904.

"Peruvian Intoxicating Plant." *Chambers's Edinburgh Journal*, no. 245 (8th October 1836): 296.

"Pharmaceutical Society of Great Britain." *The Times*, 2nd October 1901.
"Poisons and Pharmacy Act, 1908." *Supplement to the British Medical Journal*, 9th January 1909.
"Prof. Dr. Sampson's Coca Präparate." *Rhein- und Ruhrzeitung*, 2nd December 1873.
"Prof. Dr. Sampson's Coca Präparate." *Schwäbischer Merkur*, 8th July 1873.
"Schwächezustände alter und junger Männer..." *Kölnische Zeitung*, 7th January 1867.
"Scientific Intelligence. A New Stimulant." *The London Review*, 14th September 1861.
"Some Popular Remedies." *Chambers's Journal of Popular Literature, Science and Arts* 12, no. 577 (19th January 1895): 42–5.
"Suicide with Cocaine." *The Daily News*, 9th April 1896.
"Tausende, welche schon seit langer Zeit..." *Kölnische Zeitung*, 30th August 1876.
"The Charge of Poisoning." *The Times*, 31st August 1891.
"The Chymistry of Common Life." *The Times*, 20th January 1855.
"The Coca Chewers of Peru." *The London Saturday Journal* 2, no. 47 (23rd November 1839): 326–7.
"The Coca Plant." *The Times*, 18th January 1889.
"The Cocaine Cure for Sea-Sickness." *The Guardian*, 12th October 1886.
"The Coca-Leaf." *The Times*, 24th March 1876.
"The Dangers of Coca Wines." *British Medical Journal* (4th December 1897): 1666.
"The General Practitioners and the New Pharmacy Act." *Daily News*, 24th November 1868.
"The History of Coca." *The Lancet* vol. 173 issue 4459 (13th February 1909): 485.
"The Narcotics we indulge in." *Blackwood's Edinburgh Magazine* 74, no. 457 (November 1853): 605–28.
"The Opium Conference. Causes of Delay." *The Times*, 16th January 1912.
"The Opium Conference. Conclusion of an Agreement." *The Times*, 6th January 1912.
"The Opium Conference. Its Objects and Programme." *The Times*, 11th December 1911.
"The Opium Conference. Meeting at the Hague." *The Times*, 2nd December 1911.
"The Opium Convention." *The Times*, 14th February 1912.
"The Pharmacy Act of 1868." *The Lancet*, 14th November 1868.
"The Sale of an Asthma Remedy." *The Times*, 18th January 1908.
"The supposed Death from Cocaine." *The Daily News*, 14th October 1896.
"The Use of Cocaine." *The Birmingham Daily Post*, 27th December 1889.

"The Use of Cocaine." *The Morning Post*, 26th December 1889.

"The Use of Cocaine." *The Times*, 4th September 1908.

"Tonic Wine. Vinacoca Tonic Wine." *The Graphic*, 18th October 1890.

"Ueber die traurigen Folgen der Cocainomanie." *Emscher Zeitung*, 3rd November 1888.

"Ueber ein neues Mittel..." *Hannoverscher Kurier*, 14th November 1884).

"Vermischtes." *Bonner Zeitung*, 4th November 1860.

"Verschiedenes." *Arnsberger Kreisblatt*, 9th February 1856.

"Vin Mariani." *All the year round* (15th August 1891): 6.

"Vinacoca." *The Graphic*, 18th October 1890.

"Vor Nachahmungen gewarnt!" *Neues Tagblatt und General-Anzeiger für Stuttgart und Württemberg*, 8th January 1876.

"We Have More than once Called Attention." *The Times*, 28th December 1889.

"Wordsworth's Coca Leaf." *The Examiner*, 29th November 1879.

"Zur Warnung." *Hannoverscher Kurier*, 3rd December 1885.

B., Albert. "Besitzen die viel angepriesenen..." *Dresdner Nachrichten*, 17th May 1875.

Baldock, J. H. "The Abuse of Narcotics." *The Times*, 15th January 1880.

Bell, J Alexander. "The Use of Coca." *British Medical Journal* (7th March 1874): 305.

Bell Taylor, Chas. "The Dangers of Cocaine." *The Lancet*, Vol. 126, Issue 3249 (5th December 1885): 1070.

Bennett, Alexander. "The Physiological Action of Coca." *British Medical Journal* (18th April 1874): 510.

Carter, William. "The Use of Coca. IV." *British Medical Journal* (28th March 1874): 414.

Christison, Robert. "Observations on the Effects of Cuca, or Coca, the Leaves of Erythroxylon Coca." *British Medical Journal*, vol. 1 no. 800 (29th April 1876): 527–531.

Chunder Bose, Kailas. "Cocaine Intoxication and its Demoralizing Effects." *British Medical Journal* (26th April 1902): 1020–1022.

Coley, Frederic C. "Medicated Wines." *British Medical Journal* (10th September 1898): 715–716.

Crespi, Alfred J H. "Some recent scientific Advances." *The Gentleman's Magazine* (October 1889): 399.

De Havilland Hall, F. "Laryngeal Spasm Caused by Cocaine Spray." *The Lancet*, Vol. 126, Issue 3247 (21st November 1885): 946.

Doyle, Arthur Conan. "Adventures of Sherlock Holmes. Adventure VI – The Man With the Twisted Lip." *The Strand Magazine* Vol. II (Jul-Dec 1891): 623–637.

F. "The Coca Plant of Peru." *The London Reader*, 11th May 1867.

F E P. "Sale of Poisons." *The Times*, 22nd September 1856.

Fox, Fortescue. "Stimulants and Narcotics." *The Nineteenth Century: A Monthly Review* 18, no. 106 (December 1885): 923–39.

Freud, Sigmund. "Ueber Coca." *Centralblatt für die gesamte Therapie* 2 (1884): 289–314.

Garrett, I. "Sale of Poisons." *The Times*, 31st January 1872.

Hodges, Frank H. "The Dangers of Cocaine." *The Lancet*, Vol. 126, Issue 3250 (12th December 1885): 1119.

Jamieson, Alexander. "Thomas's Operation for Removal of Benign Tumour of the Female Breast." *British Medical Journal* (9th June 1888): 1216–1217.

Jeaffreson, C. S. "Dangers of Cocaine." *The Lancet*, Vol. 126, Issue 3251 (19th December 1885): 1167.

Koller, Carl. "On the Use of Cocaine for Producing Anaesthesia on the Eye." Translated by J. N. Bloom. *The Lancet*, Vol. 124, Issue 3197 (6th December 1884): 990–92.

Leared, Arthur. "The Use of Coca." *British Medical Journal* (28th February 1874): 272.

Leslie Callaghan, Jas. "The Poisonous Effects of Cocaine Taken Internally." *The Lancet*, Vol. 127, Issue 3276 (12th June 1886): 1149.

Mattison, J. B. "Cocaine Dosage and Cocaine Addiction." *The Lancet* (21st May 1887): 1024–1026.

Mivart, George. "Cocaine." *British Medical Journal* (6th December 1884): 1131.

Otto, Hans. "Warnung vor dem Cocain." *Hagener Zeitung*, 9th September 1890.

Prosser, James. "Substitutes for Cocaine." *The Lancet*, Vol. 126, Issue 3227 (4th July 1885): 10–11.

Savory and Moore. "The Use of Coca." *British Medical Journal* (28th February 1874): 289.

Seige, Max. "Klinische Erfahrungen mit Neuronal." *Deutsche medizinische Wochenschrift*, 38 (1912): 1828–30.

Sieveking, E H. "Coca: Its Therapeutic Use." *British Medical Journal* (21st February 1874): 234.

Stockman, Ralph. "Reports to the Scientific Grants Committee of the British Medical Association. Report on the Coca Alkaloids." *British Medical Journal* (11th May 1889): 1043–1046.

Sumner, W. G. "The Spanish Dollar and the Colonial Shilling." *The American Historical Review*, Vol. 3 No. 4 (Jul. 1898): 607–619.

W W. "Sale of Poisons." *The Times*, 10th October 1856.

Unpublished Sources

Personal Communication

Anderson, John. *John Anderson to the Earl of Crewe*. 30th March 1910. Letter. TNA.

Arnold, H. H. *Arnold to John Reader Jackson*. 25th July 1893. Letter. DC/163/3. Directors' Correspondence, 163 – Ceylon Letters. London: Kew Royal Botanic Gardens Archive.

Baddeley, F M. *F M Baddeley to the Colonial Secretary*. 1st June 1910. Letter.

Bidie, George. *George Bidie to Sir Joseph Dalton Hooker*. 30th April 1884. Letter. DC/157/138. Directors' Correspondence, 157 – Indian Letters Madras, Mysore. London: Kew Royal Botanic Gardens Archive.

Bidie, George. *George Bidie to Sir William Thiselton-Dyer*. 21st October 1884. Letter. DC/157/141. Directors' Correspondence, 157 – Indian Letters Madras, Mysore. London: Kew Royal Botanic Gardens Archive.

Blechynden, Richard. *Richard Blechynden to Sir Daniel Morris*. 10th April 1888. Letter. DC/153/89. Directors' Correspondence, 153 – Indian Letters Bengal, Assam, Burma. London: Kew Royal Botanic Gardens Archive.

Blechynden, Richard. *Richard Blechynden to Sir Daniel Morris*. 31st January 1888. Letter. DC/153/87. Directors' Correspondence, 153 – Indian Letters Bengal, Assam, Burma. London: Kew Royal Botanic Gardens Archive.

Broughton, John. *John Broughton to Sir Joseph Dalton Hooker*. 22nd January 1867. Letter. DC/157/149. Director's Correspondence, 157 – Indian Letters Madras, Mysore. London: Kew Royal Botanic Gardens Archive.

Burck, William. *William Burck to Daniel Morris*. 23rd February 1888. Letter. DC/165/60. Directors' Correspondence, 165 – East Asia Letters I. London: Kew Royal Botanic Gardens Archive.

Campbell, William Hunter. *William Hunter Campbell to Sir Joseph Dalton Hooker*. 22nd April 1868. Letter. DC/204/231. Directors' Correspondence, 204 – Central America & British Guiana Letters. London: Kew Royal Botanic Gardens Archive.

Consul General. *Consul General to W G Max Müller*. 11th July 1912. Letter. TNA.

Curtis, Charles. *Charles Curtis to Sir Joseph Dalton Hooker*. 14th July 1885. Letter. DC/165/174. Directors' Correspondence, 165 – East Asia Letters I. London: Kew Royal Botanic Gardens Archive.

Duff, Mountstuart Elphinstone Grant. *Mountstuart Elphinstone Grant Duff to Sir William Thiselton-Dyer*. 20th January 1885. Letter. DC/157/359. Directors'

Correspondence, 157 – Indian letters Madras, Mysore. London: Kew Royal Botanic Gardens Archive.

Dunstan, Wyndham R. "Memorandum on the Production, Distribution, Sale and Physiological Effects of Cocaine." 16th November 1909. In: H Bertram Cox to E Grey. Letter. 1st June 1910. London: TNA.

E, W. E W to A Langman. 17th September 1903. Letter. Wellcome Collection.

Edwards, E. H. E. H. *Edwards to Sir William Thiselton-Dyer*. 16th April 1884. Letter. DC/188/247. Directors' Correspondence, 188 – Mascarene Islands Letters. London: Kew Royal Botanic Gardens Archive.

Ernst, Adolf. *Adolf Ernst to Sir William Thiselton-Dyer*. 2nd February 1889. Letter. DC/215/563. Directors' Correspondence, 215 – Northern South America & Brazil Letters. London: Kew Royal Botanic Gardens Archive.

Fawcett, William. *William Fawcett to Daniel Morris*. 25th January 1889. Letter. DC/210/217. Directors' Correspondence, 210 – Jamaica Letters Arber-Harris. London: Kew Royal Botanic Gardens Archive.

Fawcett, William. *William Fawcett to Daniel Morris*. 2nd May 1892. Letter. DC/210/352. Directors' Correspondence, 210 – Jamaica Letters Arber-Harris. London: Kew Royal Botanic Gardens Archive.

Ferguson, William. *William Ferguson to Sir William Jackson Hooker*. 30th September 1850. Letter. DC/54/154. Directors' Correspondence, 54 – East Indian Letters. London: Kew Royal Botanic Gardens Archive.

Gammie, James Alexander. *James Alexander Gammie to Sir William Thiselton-Dyer*. 13th October 1890. Letter. DC/153/303. Directors' Correspondence, 153 – Indian Letters Bengal, Assam, Burma. London: Kew Royal Botanic Gardens Archive.

Gammie, James Alexander. *James Alexander Gammie to Sir William Thiselton-Dyer*. 11th April 1892. Letter. DC/153/305. Directors' Correspondence, 153 – Indian Letters Bengal, Assam, Burma. London: Kew Royal Botanic Gardens Archive.

Gray, John. *John Gray to Daniel Morris*. 13th January 1888. Letter. DC/214/370. Directors' Correspondence, 214 – Winward Islands Letters. London: Kew Royal Botanic Gardens Archive.

Hart, John Hinchley. *John Hinchley Hart to Daniel Morris*. 17th November 1887. Letter. DC/213/57. Directors' Correspondence, 213 – Trinidad & Tobago Letters. London: Kew Royal Botanic Gardens Archive.

Hartig and Calker. *Hartig and Calker to the Royal Botanic Gardens*. 16th February 1893. Letter. DC/165/73. Directors' Correspondence, 165 – East Asia Letters I. London: Kew Royal Botanic Gardens Archive.

Horne, John. *John Horne to D. Morris*. 26th October 1886. Letter. DC/188/429. Directors' Correspondence, 188 – Mascarene Island Letters. London: Kew Royal Botanic Gardens Archive.

Horne, John. *John Horne to Daniel Morris*. 7th February 1888. Letter. DC/188/435. Directors' Correspondence, 188 – Mascarene Islands Letters. London: Kew Royal Botanic Gardens Archive.

Howard, Alfred G. *Alfred G. Howard to John Reader Jackson*. 6th June 1893. Letter. DC/163/144. Directors' Correspondence, 163 – Ceylon Letters. London: Kew Royal Botanic Gardens Archive.

Howarth, Osbert H. *Osbert H. Howart to Royal Botanic Gardens*. 12th August 1885. Letter. DC/181/84. Directors' Correspondence, 181 – Atlantic Island Letters. London: Kew Royal Botanic Gardens Archive.

Howarth, Osbert H. *Osbert H. Howarth to Sir William Thiselton-Dyer*. 17th July 1885. Letter. DC/181/83. Directors' Correspondence, 181 – Atlantic Island Letters. London: Kew Royal Botanic Gardens Archive.

Jennings, Samuel. *Samuel Jennings to Sir Joseph Dalton Hooker*. 22nd January 1885. Letter. DC/153/357a. Directors' Correspondence, 153 – Indian Letters Bengal, Assam, Burma. London: Kew Royal Botanic Gardens Archive.

Jones, Joseph. *Joseph Jones to Daniel Morris*. 3rd May 1892. Letter. DC/212/267. Directors' Correspondence, 212 – Leeward Island Letters. London: Kew Royal Botanic Gardens Archive.

Key, E. Bassett. *E. Bassett Key to Daniel Morris*. 15th March 1887. Letter. DC/211/682. Directors' Correspondence, 211 – Jamaica Letters Hart-Wil. London: Kew Royal Botanic Gardens Archive.

Langley, W. *W Langley to the Under Secretary of State*. 13th May 1910. Letter. London: TNA.

Lawson, Marmaduke Alexander. *Marmaduke Alexander Lawson to Sir William Thiselton-Dyer*. 14th April 1885. Letter. DC/157/490. Directors' Correspondence, 157 – Indian Letters Madras, Mysore. London: Kew Royal Botanic Gardens Archive.

Lawson, Marmaduke Alexander. *Marmaduke Alexander Lawson to Sir William Thiselton-Dyer*. 23rd April 1885. Letter. DC/157/492. Directors' Correspondence, 157 – Indian Letters Madras, Mysore. London: Kew Royal Botanic Gardens Archive.

Lewis and Peat. *Lewis and Peat to John Reader Jackson*. 6th March 1900. Letter. DC/184/129. Directors' Correspondence, 184 – West African Letters. London: Kew Royal Botanic Gardens Archive.

Lewis and Peat. *Lewis and Peat to the Royal Botanic Gardens*. 2nd March 1900. Letter. DC/184/130. Directors' Correspondence, 184 – West African Letters. London: Kew Royal Botanic Gardens Archive.

Mathews, Andrew. *Andrew Mathews to Sir William Jackson Hooker*. 20th August 1833. Letter. DC/67/120. Directors' Correspondence, 67 – S. American Letters. London: Kew Royal Botanic Gardens Archive.

Müller, W G. *W G Max Müller Max to Earl Grey*. 19th February 1910. Letter. London: TNA.

Powell, Henry. *Henry Powell to Daniel Morris*. 6th May 1892. Letter. DC/214/520. Directors' Correspondence, 214 – Winward Islands Letters. London: Kew Royal Botanic Gardens Archive.

Thwaites, George Henry Kendrick. *George Henry Kendrick Thwaites to Sir Joseph Dalton Hooker*. 11th November 1870. Letter. DC/162/418. Directors' Correspondence, 162 – Ceylon Letters. London: Kew Royal Botanic Gardens Archive.

Trimen, Henry. *Henry Trimen to Daniel Morris*. 29th January 1889. Letter. DC/163/431. Directors' Correspondence, 163 – Ceylon Letters. London: Kew Royal Botanic Gardens Archive.

Trimen, Henry. *Henry Trimen to Sir William Thiselton-Dyer*. 13th November 1894. Letter. DC/163/521. Directors' Correspondence, 163 – Ceylon Letters. London: Kew Royal Botanic Gardens Archive.

Willis, John Christopher. *John Christopher Willis to Sir William Thiselton-Dyer*. 18th February 1902. Letter. DC/164/16. London: Kew Royal Botanic Gardens Archive.

Ephemera

"Burrough Coca Wine Chelsea Erythroxylon Coca." Leaflet. Ca. 1896. Wellcome Collection.

"Cocaine "Tabloids."." Leaflet. 27th November 1891. Burroughs, Wellcome & Co.

"Eucain Hydrochlorate." Leaflet. Ca. 1896. Burroughs, Wellcome & Co.

"Hall's Coca Wine." Leaflet. No 194: 14. Wellcome Collection.

"Hall's Coca Wine: a marvellous restorative." Advert. Ca. 1890–1899. Wellcome Collection.

"Hall's Coca Wine: the elixir of life." Advert. Ca. 1916. Wellcome Collection.

"Hall's Coca Wine is not a patent medicine." Leaflet. Ca. 1890s. Wellcome Collection.

"Hall's Wine." Leaflet. Ca. 1890. Wellcome Collection.

"Howard and Sons Limited {Chemists}." Treatise. ACC/1037. The London Archives.

"Hypodermic medication. Notes on Alkaloids. Antidote Tables and Precautions." Miniature booklet. Ca. 1890s. Burroughs & Wellcome.

"James Burrough's Coca Wine." Leaflet. Ca. 1890s. Wellcome Collection.

"The pure Aluminium hypodermic syringe." Leaflet. Ca. 1890s. Burroughs, Wellcome & Co.

"The Story of Cocaine." Treatise. 27th February 1930. Wellcome Institute.

"Verordnung." Newspaper cutting. 28th July 1910. TNA.

Angerer, -. "Carl Koller, inscribed on reverse: Seinem lieben Freund Dr Sigmund Freud. April 1885 Dr Carl Koller." Photograph. April 1885. Freud Museum, London. https://www.freud.org.uk/collections/archives/archive-records/IN/1510/.

Historiography

Books

Benson, John. *The Rise of Consumer Society in Britain, 1880–1980*. London, 1994.

Bentley, Tamara H., ed. *Picturing Commerce in and from the East Asian Maritime Circuits, 1550–1800*. Amsterdam University Press, 2019.

Berridge, Virginia and Edwards, Griffith. *Opium and the People. Opiate Use in Nineteenth-Century England*. London, New York: St. Martin's Press, 1987.

Coelsch-Foisner, Sabine und Christopher Herzog, ed. *For Sale! Kommodifizierung in der Gegenwartskultur*. Heidelberg: Universitätsverlag Winter, 2021.

Collins, Cornelius Francis. *The drug evil and the drug law*. New York: M.B. Brown, 1918.

Courtwright, David T. *Forces of Habit*. Cambridge: Harvard University Press, 2001.

Derks, Hans. *History of the Opium Problem. The Assault on the East, ca. 1600–1950*. Leiden: Brill, 2012.

Eckart, Wolfgang Uwe und Robert Jütte. Medizingeschichte. Eine Einführung. Köln: Böhlau Verlag, 2014.

Foxcroft, Louise. *The Making of Addiction: The 'Use and Abuse' of Opium in Nineteenth-Century Britain*. Burlington: Ashgate Publishing Company, 2007.

Fuhse, Jan. *Social Networks of Meaning and Communication*. Oxford: Oxford University Press, 2022.

Goodman, Jordan, Sherratt, Andrew, and Lovejoy, Paul E. Consuming Habits: Global and Historical Perspectives on How Cultures Define Drugs: Drugs in History and Anthropology. Florence: Taylor & Francis Group, 2007.

Gootenberg, Paul, ed. Cocaine: Global Histories. London: Routledge, 1999.

Gootenberg, Paul. Andean *Cocaine: The Making of a Global Drug*. Chapel Hill: The University of North Carolina Press, 2008.

Hager, Hermann. *Handbuch der pharmaceutischen Praxis*. Bd. 1. Berlin: Springer, 1876.

Hindle, Wilfrid Hope. *The Morning Post, 1772–1937: portrait of a newspaper.* London: Routledge, 1974.

Holloway, S W F. *Royal Pharmaceutical Society of Great Britain, 1841–1991, A Political and Social History.* London: The Pharmaceutical Press, 1991.

Inglis, Brian. *The Forbidden Game. A Social History of Drugs.* New York City: Charles Scribner's Sons, 1975.

Karch, Steven B. A Brief History of Cocaine. Boca Raton: CRC Press, 1998.

Kennedy, Joseph. Coca Exotica. The Illustrated Story of Cocaine. London: Associated University Presses, 1985.

Mortimer, W. Golden. *History of Coca: "The Divine Plant" of the Incas.* J. H. Vail: New York, 1901.

Parssinen, T. M. *Secret Passions, Secret Remedies. Narcotic Drugs in British Society 1820–1930.* Philadelphia: Institute for the Study of Human Issues, Inc. 1983.

Ramusack, Barbara. *The Indian Princes and their States.* Cambridge: Cambridge University Press, 2004.

Said, Edward. *Culture and Imperialism.* New York: Knopf, 1993.

Shaw, W A. *The History of Currency 1252 to 1894.* London: Clement Wilson, 1896.

Torgovnick, Marianna. *Gone Primitive: Savage Intellects, Modern Lives.* Chicago: Chicago University Press, 1990.

Book Chapters

Allen, Catherine J. "Coca and Cultural Identity in Andean Communities." In: *Coca and Cocaine. Effects on People and Policy in Latin America,* edited by Deborah Pacini and Christine Franquemont, 35–48. Peterborough: Transcript Printing Company, 1986.

Harley, C Knick. "Trade: Discovery, Mercantilism and Technology." In: *The Cambridge Economic History of Modern Britain*, edited by Roderick Floud and Paul Johnson, 175–203. Cambridge: Cambridge University Press, 2004.

Pinwinkler, Alexander. "'Assimilation' und 'Dissimilation' in der 'Bevölkerungsgeschichte', ca. 1918 bis 1960," In: *Bevölkerungsforschung und Politik in Deutschland im 20. Jahrhundert*, edited by Rainer Mackensen, 23–48. Wiesbaden: VS Verlag für Sozialwissenschaften, 2006.

Articles

Amarawat, Vikram Singh. "Cultural Imperialism and Travel Writing: Glimpses of Richard Burton's Travelogue." *Proceedings of the Indian History Congress* 77 (2016): 644–50.

Bauer, Irmgard. "Travel Medicine, Coca and Cocaine: Demystifying and Rehabilitating *Erythroxylum* – a Comprehensive Review." *Tropical Diseases, Travel Medicine and Vaccines* 5 (2019): 1–14.

Berg, Maxine. "In Pursuit of Luxury: Global History and British Consumer Goods in the Eighteenth Century." *Past & Present*, no. 182 (2004): 85–142.

Berridge, Virginia. "Morality and medical science: Concepts of narcotic addiction in Britain, 1820–1926." *Annals of Science*, Volume 36, Issue 1 (1979): 67–85.

Biondich, Amy Sue and Jeremy David Joslin. "Coca: The History and Medical Significance of an Ancient Andean Tradition." *Emergency Medicine International* (2016): 1–5.

Borgmann, Albert. "A Moral Conception of Commodification." In: Nico Stehr, Christoph Henning, Bernd Weiler, eds. *The moralization of the markets*. New York, London: Routledge, 2017: 193–210.

Boucher, Douglas H. "Cocaine and the Coca Plant." *BioScience* 41, no. 2 (1991): 72–76.

Coles, Anne-Marie. "Non-Linear Discourse and Control of Technology: The Pharmaceutical Society and Poisons Legislation in 19th-Century Britain." *Sociology* 51 (3) (2017): 511–526.

Comstock, Alzada. "British Economic Policy: I. Mercantilism." *Current History* 19, no. 109 (1950): 135–38.

Conrad, Peter and Kristin K Barker. "The Social Construction of Illness: Key Insights and Policy Implications." *Journal of Health and Social Behavior* Volume 51, Issue 1 (2010): 1–159.

Diebolt, Claude and Michael Haupert. "Cliometrics: Past, Present, and Future" *Association Francaise de Cliométrie* Nr.4 (2021): 1–18, https://hal.science/hal-03345558/document.

Gagliano, Joseph A. "The Popularization of Peruvian Coca." *Revista De Historia De América*, no. 59 (1965): 164–179.

Goerig, Michael, Douglas Bacon, and André van Zundert. "Carl Koller, Cocaine, and Local Anesthesia." *Regional Anesthesia and Pain Medicine*, Volume 37, Number 3 (2012): 318–324.

Gootenberg, Paul. "A Forgotten Case of 'Scientific Excellence on the Periphery'": The Nationalist Cocaine Science of Alfredo Bignon, 1884–1887." *Comparative Studies in Society and History* 49, no. 1 (2007): 202–32.

Gootenberg, Paul. "Talking about the Flow: Drugs, Borders, and the Discourse of Drug Control." *Cultural Critique*, no. 71 (2009): 13–46.

Heath, Wesley J. "America's First Drug Regulation Regime: The Rise and Fall of the Import Drug Act of 1848." *Food and Drug Law Journal* 59, no. 1 (2004): 169–199.

Hobbs, Andrew. "The deleterious dominance of The Times in nineteenth-century historiography." *Journal of Victorian Culture* 18 (4) (2013): 472–497.

Jay, Mike. "Miracle or Menace? The Arrival of Cocaine 1860–1900." *International Review of Neurobiology*, Volume 120 (2015): 27–39.

Karmel, Richard. "Freud's "Cocaine Papers" (1884–1887): A Commentary." *Canadian Journal of Psychoanalysis* 11, no. 1 (Spring, 2003): 161–169.

Kennedy, Dane. "British Exploration in the Nineteenth Century: A Historiographical Survey." *History Compass* 5/6 (2007): 1879–1900.

Knoblauch, Hubert. "Reflexive Methodology and the Empirical Theory of Science." *Historical Social Research / Historische Sozialforschung* 46, no. 2 (2021): 59–79.

Koster, Martijn, and Yves van Leynseele. "Brokers as Assemblers: Studying Development Through the Lens of Brokerage." *Ethnos* 83 (5) (2018): 803–13.

Majander, Kerttu, Saskia Pfrengle, Arthur Kocher, et al."Ancient bacterial genomes reveal a high diversity of Treponema pallidum Strains in early Modern Europe." *Current Biology* 30 (19) (2020): 3788 – 3803.

Mills, James H. "Cocaine and the British Empire: The Drug and the Diplomats at the Hague Opium Conference, 1911–12." *The Journal of Imperial and Commonwealth History* Vol. 42, No. 3 (2014): 400–419.

Mold, Alex. "'Consuming Habits': Histories of Drugs in Modern Societies." *Cultural & Social History* 4 (2) (2007): 261–70.

Pearce, D. N. "Sherlock Holmes, Conan Doyle and Cocaine." *Journal of the History of the Neurosciences*, 3:4 (1994): 227–232.

Plowman T and L Rivier. "Cocaine and Cinnamoylcocaine content of thirty-one species of Erythroxylum (Erythroxylaceae)." *Annals of Botany* (1983): 641–659.

Price, Richard. "One Big Thing: Britain, Its Empire, and Their Imperial Culture." *Journal of British Studies*, Vol. 45, No. 3 (July 2006): 602–627.

Reed, James. "A Medical Perspective on the Adventures of Sherlock Holmes." *Journal of Medical Ethics: Medical Humanities* 27 (2001): 76–81.

Reinsch, Paul S. "Diplomatic Affairs and International Law, 1909." *The American Political Science Review* 4, no. 1 (1910): 16–51.

Reiser, Philip. "The Drug Industry in Peru: From Sacred Leaves to Political Curse." *KAS International Reports (Konrad Adenauer Stiftung)*, 8 (2011): 7–21.

Rhonheimer, Martin. "Politisierung und Demokratiekritik: Anmerkungen Zur Geschichte des Politisierungsbegriffes." *Archiv Für Begriffsgeschichte* 29 (1985): 138–46.

Richardson, David. "The Slave Trade, Sugar, and British Economic Growth, 1748–1776." *The Journal of Interdisciplinary History* 17, no. 4 (1987): 739–69.

Sánchez-Moreno, Maria Mcfarland. "Winding Down the War on Drugs: Reevaluating Global Drug Policy." *Harvard International Review* 36, no. 4 (2015): 35–39.

Small, Douglas. "Masters of Healing: Cocaine and the Ideal of the Victorian Medical Man." *Journal of Victorian Culture*, Volume 21, Issue 1, 1 (March 2016): 3–20.

Stearns, Peter N. "Stages of Consumerism: Recent Work on the Issues of Periodization." *The Journal of Modern History* 69, no. 1 (1997): 102–17.

Stolberg, Victor B. "The Use of Coca: Prehistory, History, and Ethnography." *Journal of Ethnicity in Substance Abuse* 10, no. 2 (April 2011): 126–46.

Wahrig, Bettina. "'Fabelhafte Dinge': Arzneimittelnarrative zu Coca und Cocain im 19. Jahrhundert." *Berichte zur Wissenschaftsgeschichte* 32 (2009): 345–364.

Thesis

Erlenbusch, Lisa. "Kommodifizierung Und Ihre Grenzen. Betrachtungen zu Markt und Gerechtigkeit." MA Thesis, Karl-Franzens Universität, Graz, 2018.

Website Content

"Betäubungsmittelgesetz – BtMG, §1." https://www.gesetze-im-internet.de/btmg_1981/__1.html. Accessed 18th June 2025.

"Burbidge, Frederick William Thomas (1847–1905)." Natural History Museum on JSTOR. https://plants.jstor.org/stable/10.5555/al.ap.person.bm000150594. Accessed 18th June 2025.

"Burbidges and Company Limited Burgoyne." Science Museum Group. https://collection.sciencemuseumgroup.org.uk/people/cp111975/burgoyne-burbidges-and-company-limited. Accessed 18th June 2025.

"Daniel Hanbury." British Museum. https://www.britishmuseum.org/collection/term/BIOG229452. Accessed 18th June 2025.

"Joseph Sturge." Quakers in the World. https://www.quakersintheworld.org/quakers-in-action/285/Joseph-Sturge. Accessed 18th June 2025.

"Martius Pharmacognostic Collection." Friedrich-Alexander Universität Nürnberg-Erlangen. https://www.fau.eu/fau/history-and-remembrance/collections-and-museums/martius-pharmacognostic-collection/. Accessed 18th June 2025.

"Money." University of Nottingham. https://www.nottingham.ac.uk/manuscriptsandspecialcollections/researchguidance/weightsandmeasures/money.aspx. Accessed 18th June 2025.

"Morning Chronicle." The British Newspaper Archive. Accessed 18th June 2025. https://www.britishnewspaperarchive.co.uk/titles/morning-chronicle.

"Neue-psychoaktive-Stoffe-Gesetz (NpSG), §2." https://www.gesetze-im-internet.de/npsg/__2.html. Accessed 18th June 2025.

Altholz, Josef F. "The Warfare of Conscience with Theology." The Victorian Web. Accessed 18th June 2025. https://www.victorianweb.org/religion/altholz/a2.html.

Banerjee, J. -. Accessed 18th June 2025. http://www.victorianweb.org/history/crime/3.html.

Cooke, Simon. "Advertisements in Victorian Books and Magazines." The Victorian Web. Last amended 25th July 2019. https://victorianweb.org/victorian/art/design/advertisements/cooke.html.

Diniejko, A. "Sherlock Holmes' Addictions." Accessed 18th June 2025. http://www.victorianweb.org/authors/doyle/addiction.html.

Diniejko, A. "Victorian Drug Use." Accessed 18th June 2025. http://www.victorianweb.org/victorian/science/addiction/addiction2.html.

European Union Drugs Agency. "Kokain und Crack: Drogenprofil." Accessed 18th June 2025. https://www.euda.europa.eu/publications/drug-profiles/cocaine_de.

European Union Drugs Agency. "Understanding Europe's drug situation in 2024 – key developments (European Drug Report 2024)." Accessed 18th June 2025. https://www.euda.europa.eu/publications/european-drug-report/2024/drug-situation-in-europe-up-to-2024_en.

Knobloch, Karl. "Apotheker Ernst Wilhelm Martius und seine Söhne Carl Friedrich Philipp und Theodor Wilhelm Christian." Collegium Alexandrinum, Universität Erlangen-Nürnberg. Last amended 5th December 2009. http://www.collegium-alexandrinum.de/martius-lebenslauf.html.

Landow, G. "The Medicinal Use of Opium in England." Accessed 18th June 2025. http://www.victorianweb.org/history/empire/opiumwars/opiumwars3.html.

Langebner, Thomas. "Über Coca in der westlichen Medizin." *Deutsche Apotheker-Zeitung*. Last modified 4th June 2016. https://www.deutsche-apotheker-zeitung.de/news/artikel/2016/05/31/cocaine-coca-medical-use-pharmacopoeia-medizin/chapter:6.

Lehne, Jakob. "Arthur Conan Doyle in Wien." Wien Museum. Accessed 18th June 2025. https://magazin.wienmuseum.at/arthur-conan-doyle-in-wien.

McDonnell, J. "Life in London." Accessed 18th June 2025. http://www.victorianweb.org/books/mcdonnell/life.html.

Paul, Maria Luisa and Bryan Pietsch. "Indigenous Colombian coca company challenges Coca-Cola's trademark." *The Washington Post*. Last amended 15th September 2024, https://www.washingtonpost.com/world/2024/09/15/coca-nasa-cola-columbia-indigenous/.

Picard, Liza. "The working classes and the poor." British Library. Accessed 18th June 2025. http://www.bl.uk/victorian-britain/articles/the-working-classes-and-the-poor.

Schneider, Gerd und Christiane Toyka-Seid. "*Das junge Politik-Lexikon: Drogen*." Bundeszentrale für politische Bildung. Accessed 18th June 2025. https://www.bpb.de/kurz-knapp/lexika/das-junge-politik-lexikon/320130/drogen/.

Stephen Smith & Co. "Hall's Coca Wine: a marvellous restorative." Advert. C 1890–1899. Wellcome Collection. Accessed 18th June 2025. https://wellcomecollection.org/works/gecumam8/images?id=dbg6hvaw.

Stephen Smith & Co. "Hall's Coca Wine: the elixir of life." Advert. C 1916. Wellcome Collection. Accessed 18th June 2025. https://wellcomecollection.org/works/snfnu6yt/images?id=b3zyxvfd.

United Nations Office on Drugs and Crime. "Sixty-sixth session." Accessed 18th June 2025. https://www.unodc.org/unodc/en/commissions/CND/session/66_Session_2023/66CND_Main.html.

United Nations Office on Drugs and Crime. "The Shanghai Opium Commission." Accessed 18th June 2025. https://www.unodc.org/unodc/en/data-and-analysis/bulletin/bulletin_1959-01-01_1_page006.html.

United Nations Office on Drugs and Crime. *Special Points of Interests*. Accessed 18th June 2025. https://www.unodc.org/documents/data-and-analysis/WDR_2024/WDR_2024_SPI.pdf.

White, William L. "Race and Class in Early Anti-drug Legislation in the United States." Accessed 18th June 2025. https://www.chestnut.org/Resources/74897b96-2909-4f2a-b927-809fb765fd06/Race-and-Class-in-Early-Anti-drug-Legislation-in-the-United-States.pdf.

WikiLectures. "Routes of drug administration." Accessed 18th June 2025. https://www.wikilectures.eu/index.php?title=Routes_of_drug_administration&oldid=25063.